Basic Anatomy and Physiology

Edited & Compiled by

Dr. B.S. Shinde
M.P.Ed., M.Phil., Ph.D.,
Lecturer, Physical Education
Shivaji University,
Kolhapur (Maharashtra)

SPORTS PUBLICATION
7/26, Ground Floor, Ansari Road,
Darya Ganj, New Delhi-110002
Phones: (Office) 65749511 (Fax) 011-23240261
(Mobile) 9868028838 (Residence) 27562163
E-mail: lakshaythani@hotmail.com

Published by:

SPORTS PUBLICATION
7/26, Ground Floor, Ansari Road, Darya Ganj, New Delhi-110002
Ph. : (Office) 65749511, 23240261 (Mobile) 9868028838
          (Residence) 27562163 (Fax) 011-23240261
E-mail: *lakshaythani@hotmail.com*

© 2010 Publishers

I.S.B.N: 978-81-7879-562-1

PRINTED IN INDIA 2010

All Rights Reserved

No part of this publication may be stored in a retrieval system, transmitted, or reproduced in any way, including but not limited to photocopy, photograph, magnetic or other record, without the prior agreement and written permission of the publisher.

Laser Typeset by:
JAIN MEDIA GRAPHICS,

Printer :
Vishal Kaushik Printers

Price: Rs. 495/-

CONTENTS

1. An Introduction to Human Anatomy   1-22
- Kinds of Anatomical Studies   2
- Organization of the Human Body   2
- Regions of the Human Body   3
- Study   5
- Regional Groups   6
- Major Organ Systems   7
- Superficial Anatomy   8
- Systems   10
- Bones   15
- The Structure of the Body   17
- The Skeleton   20

2. Basic Anatomy and Physiology   23-33
- Surface Anatomy   23
- The Skeleton   24
- The Nervous System   24
- The Respiratory System   27
- The Lungs   28
- The Circulatory System   29
- The Heart   29
- The Blood Vessels   30

- The Abdomen   32
- The Skin   33

3. The Cells and Tissues   34-60
- The Cells Organs   35
- The Cell Nucleus   36
- Components of Cells   39
- Process of Cell Division   51
- Tissues   54
- The Nucleus   59
- Cell Inclusion   60

4. Bones, Joints and Skeletal System   61-74
- Bones   61
- Functions   62
- Individual Bone Structure   63
- The Joints   65
- The Skeletal System   67
- The Skull   68
- The Pelvic Girdle and Leg   71
- The Ribs   72

5. Nervous System   75-111
- Neuro–Transmitters   76
- Neurons   76
- The Brain   78
- The Cellular Structure of the Nervous System   81

- The Nerve Centre 87
- The Nerves 88
- The Visual Area 91
- The Association Areas or Integrating Areas 96
- Localized and Unlocalized Brain Functions 97
- Maturation and Exercise in the Development of the Nervous System 98
- The Reflex Arc 99
- The Autonomic Nervous System 103

6. Circulatory System   **112-124**
- Pulmonary Circulation 114
- Systemic Circulation 114
- Coronary Circulation 114
- Heart 115
- Closed Cardiovascular System 117
- Other Vertebrates 118
- Open Circulatory System 119
- Absence of Circulatory System 120
- Measurement Techniques 120

7. Respiratory System   **125-149**
- Mucus 128
- Cilia 129
- Length 129
- Protection 129
- Ventilation and Perfusion 130

- Mechanism of Breathing 130
- Problems 133
- The Design of the Respiratory System 134
- The Pharynx 137
- The Larynx 138
- The Trachea and the Stem Bronchi 141
- Structural Design of the Airway Tree 142
- The Lungs 143
- Control of Breathing 145
- The Mechanics of Breathing 147
- Gas Exchange 148

8. Endocrine and Excretory System 150-169
- Endocrine System 150
- Function of the Endocrine System—The Nature of Endocrine Regulation 152
- Adrenal Glands 157
- Ovaries 158
- Pancreas 159
- Excretory System 161
- Excretory Functions 161
- Component Organs 162
- Physiology of the Urinary System 164

9. Digestive System 170-182
- Organization of the Digestive Tract 171
- The Mouth 173

–	The Pharynx and Oesophagus	175
–	The Small Intestine and Large Intestine	176
–	The Pancreas	179
–	The Stomach	179
–	The Liver and Gallbladder	180
–	The Physiology of Digestion	181
10.	**Sensory Systems**	**183-216**
–	Stimulus	183
–	Modality	184
–	V1 (Vision)	184
–	A1 (Auditory - Hearing)	184
–	Tongue	185
–	Visual System	185
	– Biology of the Visual System	186
	– Retina	187
	– Photochemistry	189
–	Auditory System	193
	– Ear	193
	– Neurons	197
–	Central Auditory System	197
–	Taste	199
–	Basic Tastes	201
–	Olfaction	206
–	Somatosensory System	212

11.	**Reproductive System**	**217-222**
–	Male Reproductive System	217
–	Female Reproductive System	219
12.	**Physiology of Exercise**	**223-235**
–	Effect of Exercise on Circulatory System	223
–	Effect of Exercise on Respiratory System	225
–	Effect of Exercise on Digestive System	227
–	Effect of Exercise on Skeletal System	228

1

An Introduction to Human Anatomy

    a. Anatomy is the study of the structure of the body. Often, you may be more interested in functions of the body. Functions include digestion, respiration, circulation, and reproduction. Physiology is the study of the functions of the body.

    b. The body is a chemical and physical machine. As such, it is subject to certain laws. These are sometimes called natural laws. Each part of the body is engineered to do a particular job. These jobs are functions. For each job or body function, there is a particular structure engineered to do it.

    No two human beings are built exactly alike, but we can group individuals into three major categories. These groups represent basic body shapes.

    MORPH = body, body form

    ECTO = all energy is outgoing

    ENDO = all energy is stored inside

    MESO = between, in the middle

    ECTOMORPH = slim individual

    ENDOMORPH = broad individual

    MESOMORPH = body type between the two others,

"muscular" type.

Ectomorphs, slim persons, are more susceptible to lung infections. Endomorphs are more susceptible to heart disease.

KINDS OF ANATOMICAL STUDIES

a. Microscopic anatomy is the study of structures that cannot be seen with the unaided eye. You need a microscope.

b. Gross anatomy by systems is the study of organ systems, such as the respiratory system or the digestive system.

c. Gross anatomy by regions considers anatomy in terms of regions such as the trunk, upper member, or lower member.

d. Neuroanatomy studies the nervous system.

e. Functional anatomy is the study of relationships between functions and structures.

ORGANIZATION OF THE HUMAN BODY

The human body is organized into cells, tissues, organs, organ systems, and the total organism.

a. Cells are the smallest living unit of body construction.

b. A tissue is a grouping of like cells working together. Examples are muscle tissue and nervous tissue.

c. An organ is a structure composed of several different tissues performing a particular function. Examples include the lungs and the heart.

d. Organ systems are groups of organs which together perform an overall function. Examples are the

An Introduction to Human Anatomy

respiratory system and the digestive system.

e. The total organism is the individual human being. You are a total organism.

REGIONS OF THE HUMAN BODY

The human body is a single, total composite. Everything works together. Each part acts in association with ALL other parts. Yet, it is also a series of regions. Each region is responsible for certain body activities. These regions are:

a. Back and Trunk. The torso includes the back and trunk. The trunk includes the thorax (chest) and

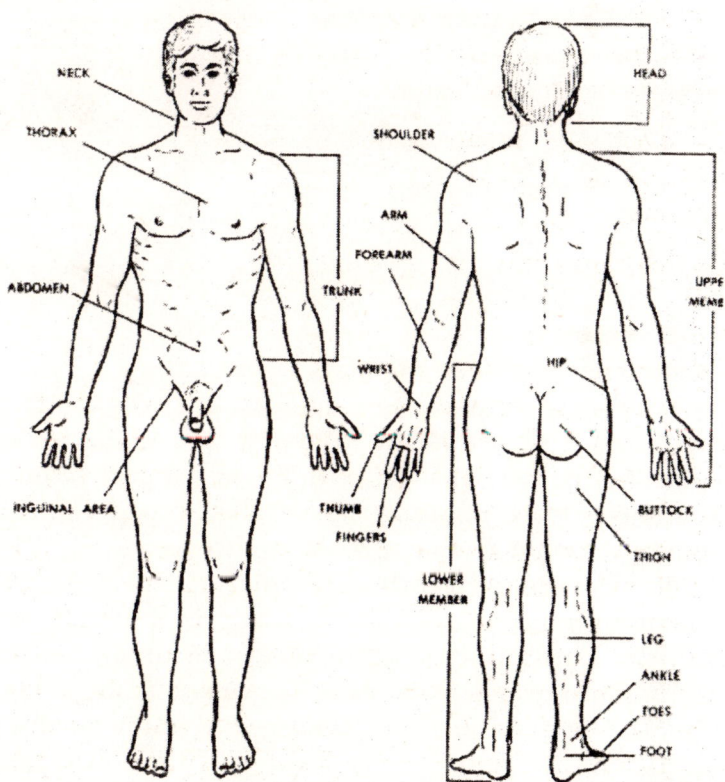

abdomen. At the lower end of the trunk is the pelvis. The perineum is the portion of the body forming the floor of the pelvis. The lungs, the heart, and the digestive system are found in the trunk.

    b. Head and Neck. The brain, eyes, ears, mouth, pharynx, and larynx are found in this region.

    c. Members.

    (1) Each upper member includes a shoulder, arm, forearm, wrist, and hand.

    (2) Each lower member includes a hip, thigh, leg, ankle, and foot.

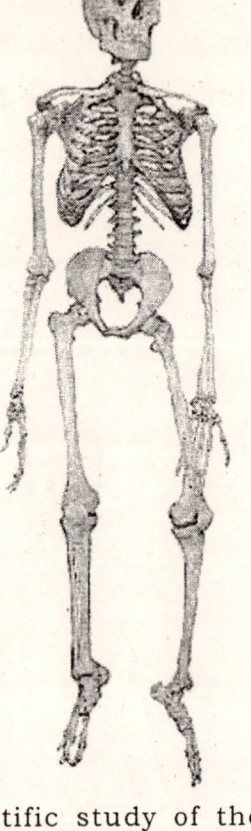

    Human anatomy, which, with physiology and biochemistry, is a complementary basic medical science is primarily the scientific study of the morphology of the adult human body. Anatomy is subdivided into gross anatomy and microscopic anatomy. Gross anatomy (also called topographical anatomy, regional anatomy, or anthropotomy) is the study of anatomical structures that can be seen by unaided vision. Microscopic anatomy is the study of minute anatomical structures assisted with microscopes, which includes histology (the study of the organization of tissues), and cytology (the study of cells). Anatomy, physiology (the study of function) and biochemistry (the study of the chemistry of living structures) are complementary basic medical sciences which are usually taught together (or in tandem).

In some of its facets human anatomy is closely related to embryology, comparative anatomy and comparative embryology, through common roots in evolution; for example, much of the human body maintains the ancient segmental pattern that is present in all vertebrates with basic units being repeated, which is particularly obvious in the vertebral column and in the ribcage, and can be traced from very early embryos.

The human body consists of biological systems, that consist of organs, that consist of tissues, that consist of cells and connective tissue.

The history of anatomy has been characterized, over a long period of time, by a continually developing understanding of the functions of organs and structures in the body. Methods have also advanced dramatically, advancing from examination of animals through dissection of preserved cadavers (dead human bodies) to technologically complex techniques developed in the 20th century.

STUDY

A full articulated human skeleton used in educationGenerally, physicians, dentists, physiotherapists, nurses, paramedics, radiographers, artists, and students of certain biological sciences, learn gross anatomy and microscopic anatomy from anatomical models, skeletons, textbooks, diagrams, photographs, lectures, and tutorials. The study of microscopic anatomy (or histology) can be aided by practical experience examining histological preparations (or slides) under a microscope; and in addition, medical and dental students generally also learn anatomy with practical experience of dissection and inspection of cadavers (dead human bodies). A thorough working knowledge of anatomy is required by all medical doctors, especially surgeons, and doctors working in some diagnostic specialities, such as histopathology and radiology.

Human anatomy, physiology, and biochemistry are basic medical sciences, which are generally taught to medical students in their first year at medical school. Human anatomy can be taught regionally or systemically; that is, respectively, studying anatomy by bodily regions such as the head and chest, or studying by specific systems, such as the nervous or respiratory systems. The major anatomy textbook, Gray's Anatomy, has recently been reorganized from a systems format to a regional format, in line with modern teaching methods.

REGIONAL GROUPS

Head and neck — includes everything above the thoracic inlet

Upper limb — includes the hand, wrist, forearm, elbow, arm, and shoulder.

Thorax — the region of the chest from the thoracic inlet to the thoracic diaphragm.

Human abdomen to the pelvic brim or to the pelvic inlet.

The back — the spine and its components, the vertebrae, sacrum, coccyx, and intervertebral disks

Pelvis and Perineum — the pelvis consists of everything from the pelvic inlet to the pelvic diaphragm. The perineum is the region between the sex organs and the anus.

Lower limb — everything below the inguinal ligament, including the hip, the thigh, the knee, the leg, the ankle, and the foot.

MAJOR ORGAN SYSTEMS

Circulatory system: pumping and channeling blood to and from the body and lungs with heart, blood, and blood vessels.

Digestive System: digestion and processing food with salivary glands, esophagus, stomach, liver, gallbladder, pancreas, intestines, rectum, and anus.

Endocrine system: communication within the body using hormones made by endocrine glands such as the hypothalamus, pituitary or pituitary gland, pineal body or pineal gland, thyroid, parathyroids, and adrenals or adrenal glands

Integumentary System: Skin, Hair and Nails

Immune system: the system that fights off disease; composed of leukocytes, tonsils, adenoids, thymus, and spleen.

Lymphatic system: structures involved in the transfer of lymph between tissues and the blood stream, the lymph and the nodes and vessels that transport it.

Musculoskeletal system: movement with muscles and human skeleton (structural support and protection with bones, cartilage, ligaments, and tendons).

Muscular system: the system that moves the body with muscles, ligaments, and tendons.

Nervous system: collecting, transferring and processing information with brain, spinal cord, peripheral nerves, and nerves

Reproductive system: the sex organs; in the female; ovaries, fallopian tubes, uterus, vagina, mammary glands, and in the male; testes, vas deferens, seminal vesicles, prostate, and penis.

Respiratory system: the organs used for breathing, the pharynx, larynx, trachea, bronchi, lungs, and diaphragm.

Skeletal system: the system that holds the body together and gives it shape; composed of bones, cartilage, and tendons.

Urinary system: kidneys, ureters, bladder and urethra involved in fluid balance, electrolyte balance and excretion of urine.

SUPERFICIAL ANATOMY

Superficial anatomy of female and male humanSuperficial anatomy or surface anatomy is important in human anatomy being the study of anatomical landmarks that can be readily identified from the contours or other reference points on the surface of the body. With knowledge of superficial anatomy, physicians gauge the position and anatomy of the associated deeper structures.

Common names of well known parts of the human body, from top to bottom:

Head — Forehead — Jaw — Cheek — Chin

Neck — Shoulders

Arm — Elbow — Wrist — Hand — Fingers — Thumb

Spine — Chest — Thorax

Abdomen — Groin

Hip — Buttocks — Leg — Thigh — Knee — Calf —

An Introduction to Human Anatomy

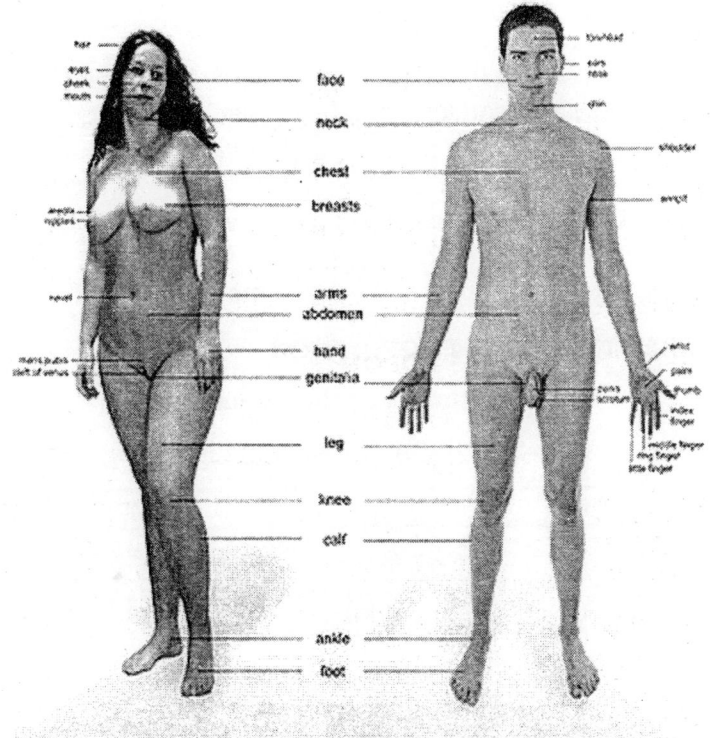

Heel — Ankle — Foot — Toes

The eye, ear, nose, mouth, teeth, tongue, throat, adam's apple, breast, penis, scrotum, clitoris, vulva, navel are also superficial structures.

Internal Organs

Common names of internal organs (in alphabetical order) :

Adrenals — Appendix — Bladder — Brain — Eyes — Gall bladder — Heart — Intestines — Kidney — Liver — Lungs — Esophagus — Ovaries — Pancreas — Parathyroids — Pituitary — Prostate — Spleen — Stomach — Testicles — Thymus — Thyroid — Uterus —

Veins.

The human body is the entire structure of a human organism, and consists of a head, neck, torso, two arms and two legs. By the time the human reaches adulthood, the body consists of close to 10 trillion cells, the basic unit of life. Groups of cells combine and work in tandem to form tissue, which combines to form organs, which work together to form organ systems.

SIZE, TYPE AND PROPORTION

Constituents of the human body

In a normal man weighing 60kg

Constituent	Weight	Percent of atoms
Oxygen	38,8 kg	25.5 %
Carbon	10.9 kg	9.5 %
Hydrogen	6.0 kg	63 %
Nitrogen	1.9 kg	1.4 %

The average height (in developed countries) of an adult male human is about 1.7–1.8 m (5'7" to 5'11") tall and the adult female about 1.6–1.7 m (5'3" to 5'7") tall. This size is firstly determined by genes and secondly by diet. Body type and body composition are influenced by postnatal factors such as diet and exercise.

SYSTEMS

The organ systems of the body include the musculoskeletal system, cardiovascular system, digestive system, endocrine system, integumentary system, urinary system, lymphatic system, immune system, respiratory system, nervous system and reproductive system.

An Introduction to Human Anatomy

Musculoskeletal System

The human musculoskeletal system consists of the human skeleton, made by bones attached to other bones with joints, and skeletal muscle attached to the skeleton by tendons.

Cardiovascular System

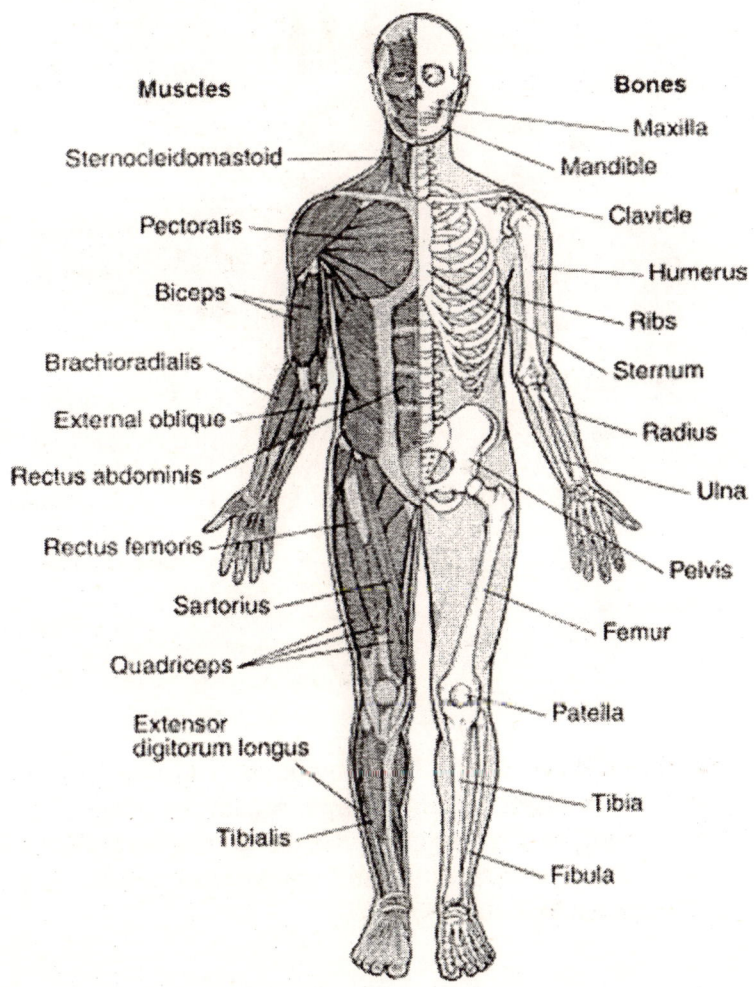

The cardiovascular system comprises the heart, veins, arteries and capillaries. The primary function of the heart is to circulate the blood, and through the blood, oxygen and vital minerals to the tissues and organs that comprise the body. The left side of the main organ (left ventricle and left atrium) is responsible for pumping

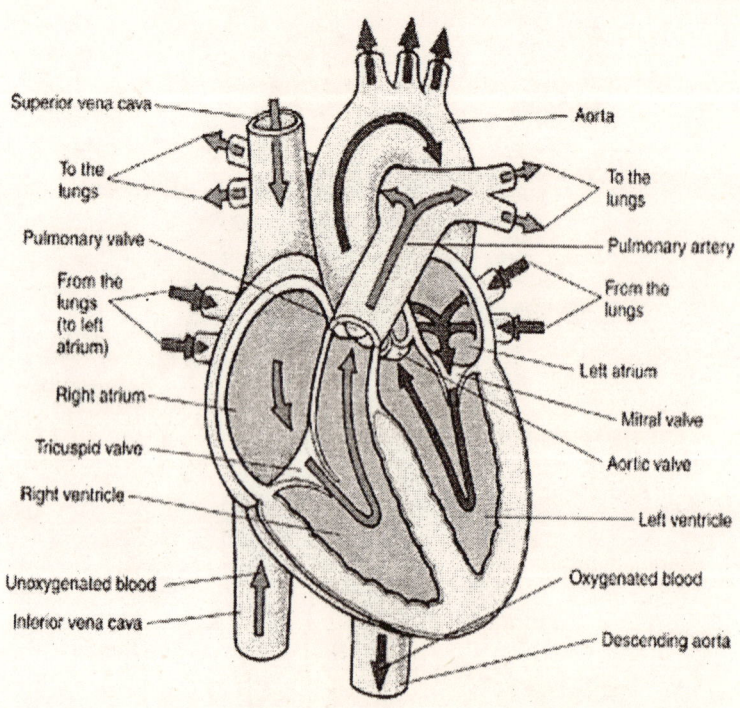

blood to all parts of the body, while the right side (right ventricle and right atrium pumps only to the lungs. The heart itself is divided into three layers called the endocardium, myocardium and epicardium, which vary in thickness and function.

An Introduction to Human Anatomy

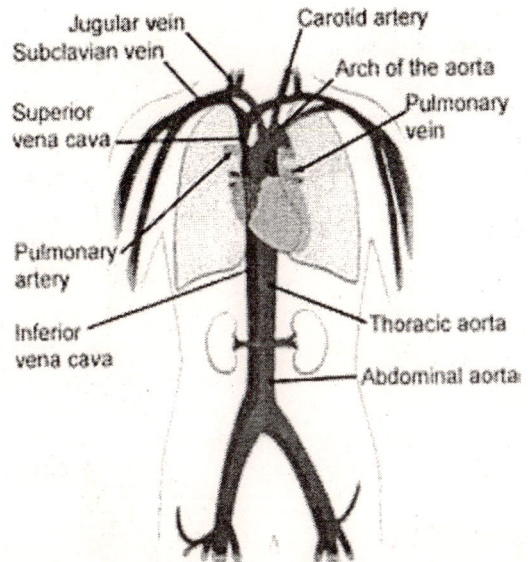

Reproductive System

Human reproduction takes place as internal fertilization by sexual intercourse. During this process, the erect penis of the male is inserted into the female's vagina until the male ejaculates semen, which contains sperm, into the female's vagina. The sperm then travels through the vagina and cervix into the uterus or fallopian tubes for fertilization of the ovum.

The human male reproductive system is a series of organs located outside the body and around the pelvic region of a male that contribute towards the reproductive process. The primary direct function of the male reproductive system is to provide the male gamete or spermatozoa for fertilization of the ovum.

The major reproductive organs of the male can be grouped into three categories. The first category is sperm production and storage. Production takes place in the testes which are housed in the temperature regulating

Basic Anatomy and Physiology

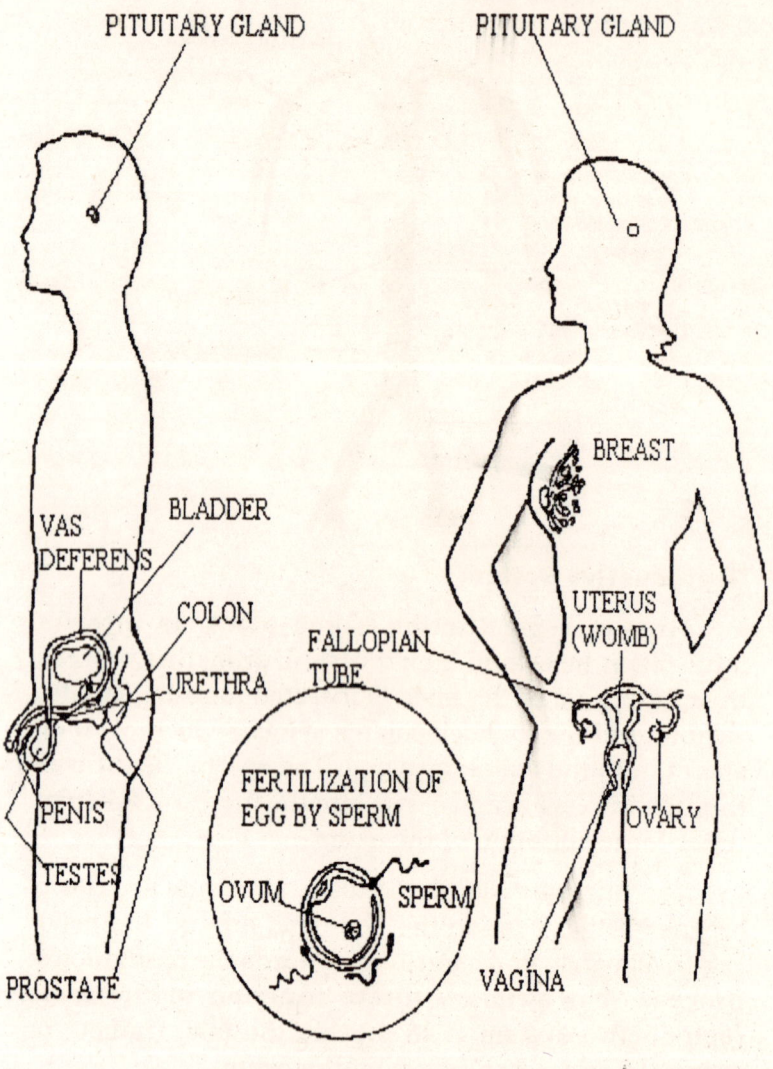

scrotum, immature sperm then travel to the epididymis for development and storage. The second category are the ejaculatory fluid producing glands which include the seminal vesicles, prostate, and the vas deferens. The final category are those used for copulation, and deposition of the spermatozoa (sperm) within the female, these include the penis, urethra, vas deferens and Cowper's gland.

The human female reproductive system is a series of organs primarily located inside of the body and around the pelvic region of a female that contribute towards the reproductive process. The human female reproductive system contains three main parts: the vagina, which acts as the receptacle for the male's sperm, the uterus, which holds the developing fetus, and the ovaries, which produce the female's ova. The breasts are also an important reproductive organ during the parenting stage of reproduction.

The vagina meets the outside at the vulva, which also includes the labia, clitoris and urethra; during intercourse this area is lubricated by mucus secreted by the Bartholin's glands. The vagina is attached to the uterus through the cervix, while the uterus is attached to the ovaries via the fallopian tubes. At certain intervals, typically approximately every 28 days, the ovaries release an ovum, which passes through the fallopian tube into the uterus. The lining of the uterus, called the endometrium, and unfertilized ova are shed each cycle through a process known as menstruation.

BONES

An adult skeleton consists of approximately 206 distinct bones:
Spine and vertebral column (26)
Cranium (8)
Face (14)
Hyoid bone, sternum and ribs (26)
Upper extremities (64)

Lower extremities (62)

But when you are first born you have over 300 bones then the bones slowly join into 206 rarely will anyone have more though.

The Whole Body

The systems that make the body work are all interdependent. This is sometimes difficult to remember when it is a matter of convenience to study each system separately. It makes learning about them easier, but it is just as possible to approach the body in a different, unconventional manner.

Little is known of how people develop is individual with their own physical and psychological differences. Some of these are the result of inheritance; clearly much is due to immediate family, and from reactions are notoriously difficult to measure; even intelligence tests are often inaccurate and may provide little indication of the brain's power of original thinking.

However, the study of a particular protein will tell a great deal about how the body functions normally. Its reaction with the digestive juices breaks it into the constituent parts, amino-acids which are than absorbed through the intestine wall and into the blood stream to the liver. In the liver the amino-acids may be rebuilt into new proteins or sent by the arterial system to help replace old proteins, such as those in muscle or reins, such as those in muscle or bone. These "worn out" amino-acids are removed form the tissues by the venous system and returned to the liver. Here they can be rebuilt or broken down into urea; urea is excreted by the kidneys into the urine.

This unconventional way of learning teaches how the digestive tract, circulation, muscle and metabolism work, but could easily involve the hormones from the endocrine system, which help instruct the body, or the nervous system, where protein may be required.

A great deal is now known about how the brain controls the other system of the body, either through quick direct nervous response or secretion of chemicals-hormones-to produce a slower reaction. The way in which the balance of salts in the blood is maintained by foods that are eaten is understood. All these physical occurrences can be watched and measured with accuracy.

THE STRUCTURE OF THE BODY

A general description—The body as a whole is a compromise between rigidity and mobility. The internal organs are closely packed together and yet can work freely and easily. The surrounding framework of bone and muscles applies support and protection.

The skeleton gives the upright strength to the body and in some places, such as the skull and thorax, acts as a protective layer. The joints give the bones mobility and the muscles strength and suppleness.

The contents of the chest and abdomen are constantly moving the beating of the heart, inspiration and expiration in the lungs and peristalsis of the bowel. These structures can move without difficulty as they are surrounded by special, smooth layers of tissue known as pericardium, pleura and peritoneum. These small cavities of tissue, or sacs to give them their medical name, are rather like a very soft balloon containing a little fluid. Push a clenched fist in one side of a balloon, press the balloon against the palm of the other hand; the moves easily and without friction. Similar "sacs" occur in the joints, around tendons passing over joints and at the points of friction, such as the knee and elbow. These are known as synovial sacs.

The body's largest organ is the skin. In an adult it covers approximately 2 square meters and not only envelops the whole body in a protective waterproof layer but is also part of the heat-regulating system. The liver, meanwhile is the most complicated organ with the greatest number of functions—transforming digested food into usable materials and disposing of waste substances.

The circulation is constantly restoring and revitalization a well as removing waste products from the basic unit of the body - the cell. The cell is a microscopic structure of which there are billions that build up the whole body. Each cell specializes and carries out its own particular function. All the structures and organs are held together by the connective tissue, made up of cells that act as a kind of packing to protect and support the internal mechanisms.

Connective Tissue—The skeleton keeps the organs, blood vessels and nerves in place and to a certain extent, provide some protection. The connective tissue supports and binds them together. It also supplies the ligaments and tendons for the joints and muscles, the tethering for the larger organs, the softness for protection and rigidity in the form of cartilage.

There are many forms of connective tissue, but they are all developed from the same jelly-like ground substance, made up of salts and water, protein and carbohydrate. Embedded in this jelly are the various fibres and cells; elastic fibres to provide elasticity; collagen fibres to provide support; white cells and macrophages to fight infection; fat cells used for storage; and finally plasma cells to produce antibodies.

Tendons and Ligaments— The strongest connective tissue is found in the tendons and ligaments. These are made of densely packed collagen fibres and may be very thick, as in the Achilles tendon, or thin and wide, as in the thin sheet of the aponeurosis that covers the skull and into which many of the skull muscles are inserted. They have to resist the pull of muscles and mobility of joints with suppleness and strength, without elasticity.

Areolar Tissue— The proportion of the different types of fibre in the ground substance gives the connective tissue its variable characteristics.

Areolar tissue is formed throughout the body in loose sheets around blood vessels, nerves and tendons; as a soft, pliable substance it helps to fill the spaces between larger organs. The tissue is made of a mixture of collagen, elastic and reticulin fibres. Under the skin and face it contains a large amount of mobile, elastic fibres, in contrast to the palms of the hands and soles of the feet, which are tough and contain more collagen fibres.

Connective tissue is found holding the cells together within organs. This can be seen in the liver, where the bile ducts, veins and arteries are held within the liver substance and in the artery wall itself; here the circular muscle is held in place by a protective sheath of loose areolar tissue. Certain diseases known as collagen diseases can afflict connective tissue, causing disorder of their normal function. The skin becomes wrinkled and creased with age as the elastic fibres degenerate. This occurs more rapidly when they are damaged by ultraviolet sunlight which is partly prevented by more pigmentation.

Cartilage— Cartilage is a special form of connective tissue and supplies the fabric for the formation of bone. Bone forms by ossification—the process by which minute crystals of calcium salts are manufactured by osteoblast cells and arranged in layers.

Adult cartilage does not contain blood vessels or nerves but is filled with small holes to allow nutrition to seep into it. There are three forms of cartilage: Elastic cartilage is mainly densely packed cells to give it the kind of springiness found in the ear; fibro-cartilage is tough and contains many more collagen fibres (the intervertebral disc of the spine has a thick circle of fibro-cartilage around the softer centre of dense connective tissue, the nucleus polypuses); and hard hyaline cartilage, found at the bone ends and in the nose, is made of dense collagen fibre.

Fat cells— The fat cells have three functions: Store, insulation, protection over certain areas, such as the buttocks, and around various organs, such as the kidneys and heart and in the liver.

Some of the areas of the body consist mainly of fat storage cells. Fat cells develop in infancy and then their total number remains constant for the rest of life. Fat babies become fat adults.

The Skeleton

Basic facts—The skeleton consists of about 206 bones divided into two broad groups, the axial and appendicular skeletons. It has three functions—it supplies support, it protects the internal organs and by using muscles, it gives movement. The axial skeleton, consisting of the skull, spine and rib cage, supplies the basic structure on to which the limbs, the appendicular skeleton, are joined via the pelvic and shoulder girdles.

Appendicular skeleton-upper limb—The shoulder girdle consists of two bones, the clavicle and scapula. The clavicle acts as a strut with one end fixed against the manubrium sterni while the outer end holds the scapula from the thorax. The glenoid cavity is for the joint with the humerus.

The arm consists of long bones and a highly mobile hand. The humerus joins the radius and ulna at the elbow and the mobility of these two bones allows pronation and supination of the forearm and hand.

Appendicular skeleton-lower limb—The pelvis is much stronger than the shoulder girdle because it has support the full weight of the body. Each innominate is formed from 3 bones - the wing-shaped ilium, the pubis in front and the ischium behind. These are fused together. In front the innominate bones articulate at the symphysis pubis and join the massive sacrum behind. All these 3 bones form the acetabulum for the articulation of the femur.

The lower and upper limbs are similar but with different functions. The long femur has its head extended to the side by the neck to articulate in the acetabulum. Large tubercles-the greater and lesser trochanters - are formed for muscle insertion. The lower end of the femur articulates the tibia, with the patella in front; the fibula supplies support for the muscles and part of the ankle joint. The 7 tarsals and 5 metatarsals support the body weight; the 14 phalanges are much smaller in the hand as they have little active function.

Axial skeleton- spine— The spine consists of 7 cervical, 12 thoracic and 5 lumbar vertebrae. The 5 sacral and 4 vertebrae of the coccyx fuse together to make solid bone.

Axial skeleton - thorax— The thorax consists of 12 pairs of bibs, articulating with the thoracic vertebrae, 10 pairs joined with cartilaginous processes to the sternum in front leaving the two lowest pairs floating. The sternum consists of the manubrium, at the top, and the small xiphi-stermum at the lower end. Some people have an extra vertebra or an extra rib.

Bone structure— All bones have an outer, compact, dense layer and inner, spongy, cancellous centre. This makes them strong but light. Bones also store calcium and phosphorus and in many the cancellous centre is replaced by a medulla containing the marrow - blood-forming cells-or, in the case of sinuses, in air-containing space.

The articular surfaces of bone are covered with cartilage to supply a smooth surface for the joint. The overall surface of most bones is irregular and grooved by blood vessels or nerves. Bones are surrounded by tough, fibrous periosteum into which muscles and ligaments are inserted. Their traction causes ridges, tubercles or crests to occur by periosteal reaction - new bone formation. There is no nerve supply to bone, but blood vessels enter through the nutrient canal to reach the cancellous centre.

Bone growth — Growth takes place in all bones, but is more obviously apparent in the long bones. An infant's long bones have bony ends - epiphyses-separated from the shaft by the cartilagenous dis-physical line of new bone formation. By the age of 25 (earlier in women) all these diaphyseal lines have ceased growing and have fused with the bone. Short and irregular bones, like carpal bones and the maxilla, calcify from the centre. Flat bones start as a membranous sheet that forms bone and gradually thickens to a centre of cancellous bones.

2

Basic Anatomy And Physiology

SURFACE ANATOMY

Surface anatomy is the identification of landmarks on the surface of the skin allows us to compare our knowledge of our own surface anatomy with that of an injured person. The best way to learn about surface anatomy is to look at and examine your own body. What you learn from this will help you find injuries on others.

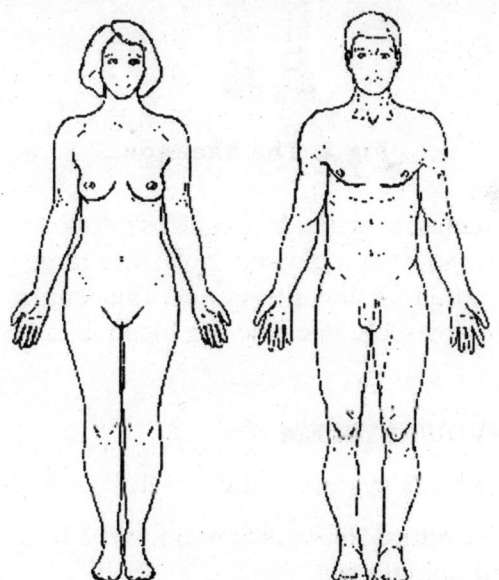

Fig 1: Male and female adults in the anatomical position

THE SKELETON

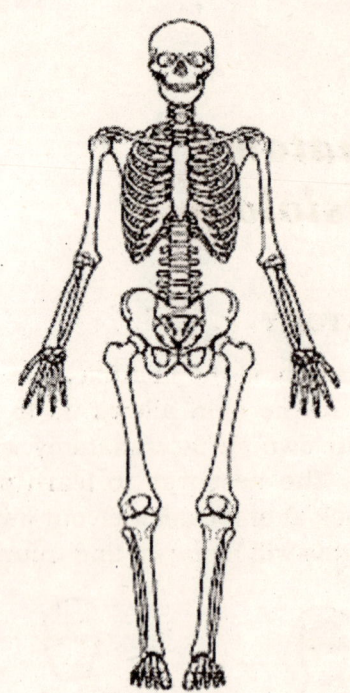

Fig 2: The Skeleton

The skeleton is made up of bone which is living tissue that requires a blood supply. The larger bones in the body, such as the pelvis and the femurs, have a greater blood supply because the blood is made in their marrow.

THE NERVOUS SYSTEM

The nervous system is divided into three parts:

1. The Central Nervous System of the brain, cranial nerves and spinal cord;

BrainSpinal Cord

Basic Anatomy and Physiology 25

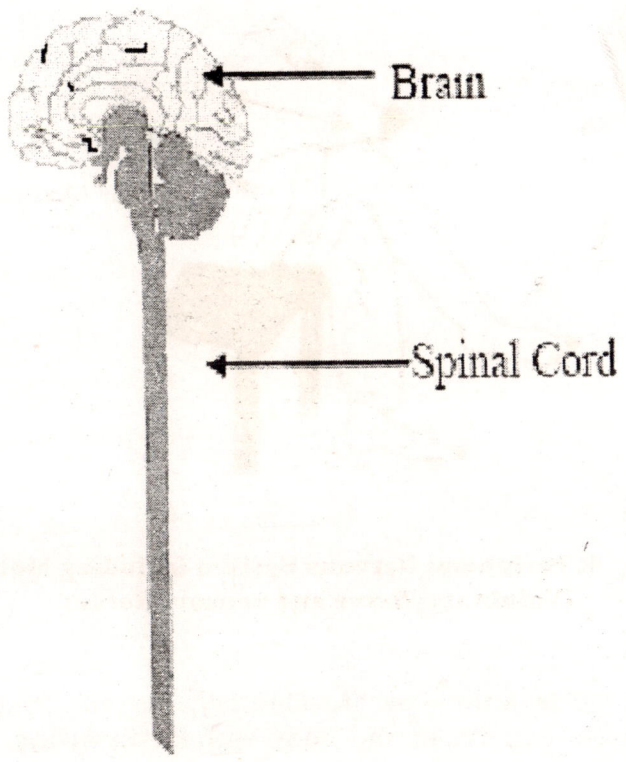

Fig. 3: The Central Nervous System

2. The Peripheral Nervous System comprising motor (voluntary) nerves and sensory nerves. The brain uses motor (voluntary) nerves to transmit commands to the muscles so when you wish to pick up a glass the motor nerves tell the muscles of the hand, arm, shoulder and chest to move.

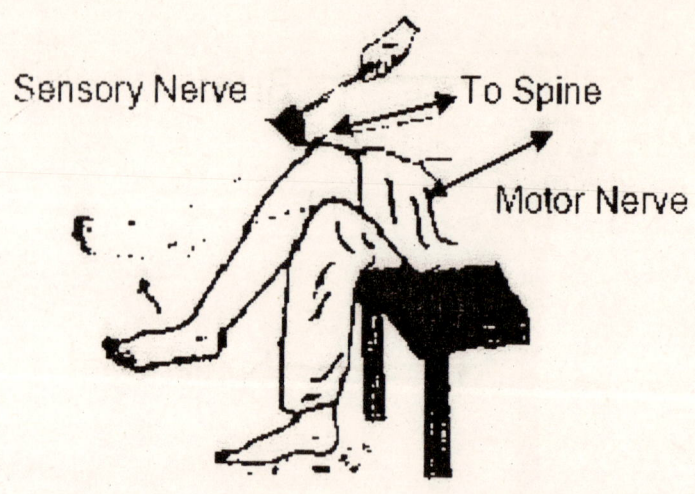

Fig. 4: Peripheral Nervous System including Motor (Voluntary) Nerve and Sensory Nerves

3. The Autonomic (involuntary) Nervous System controls activity in the body without involving the conscious mind. Most of the functioning of the body is controlled by the autonomic or involuntary nervous system.

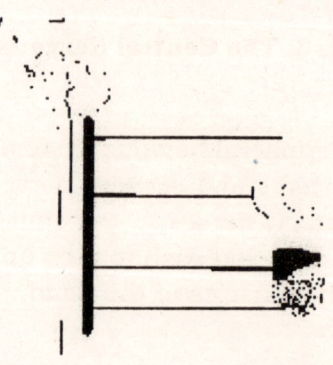

Fig. 5: Autonomic Nervous System

THE RESPIRATORY SYSTEM

The respiratory system consists of the airway, lungs and the ribs and muscles of respiration.

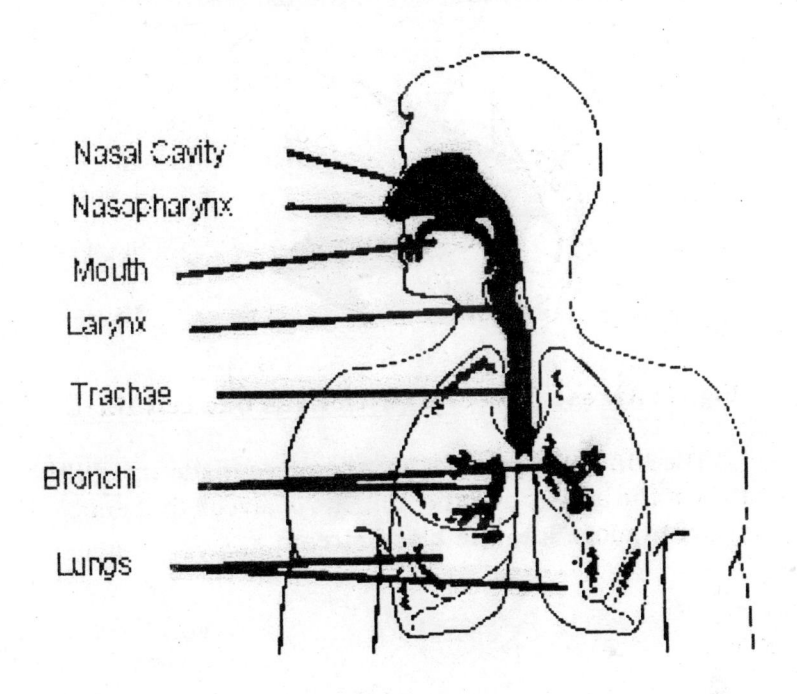

Fig. 6: The Airway

The airway extends from the lips and nostrils, through the nasal and oral cavities to the naso-pharynx and pharynx, through the larynx, tracheae, bronchi and down to the surface of the air sacs in the lungs. The airway can be blocked at any point along its length. The most common causes of such blockage are our own position, vomit, food, saliva, and blood.

THE LUNGS

The air sacs (alveoli) in the lungs are structures one cell thick. They are thin so as oxygen and other gasses can easily pass into and out of the blood stream.

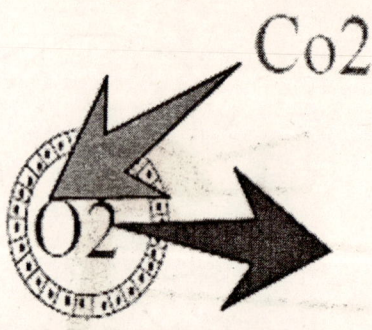

Fig. 7: Air sac (Alveolus) with walls one cell thick

The lungs themselves are therefore made up of the tubes of the airway and the millions of alveoli that enable oxygen to move into the blood stream.

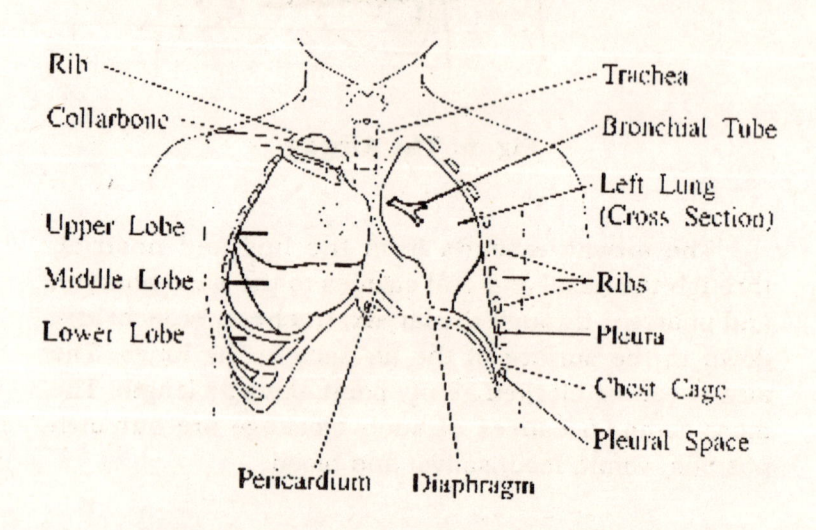

Fig. 8: The lungs and chest cavity

Basic Anatomy and Physiology

The lungs are contained within the chest and are protected by the chest wall and a layer of tough tissue called the pleurae.

THE CIRCULATORY SYSTEM

The circulatory system comprises the blood, heart, arteries, veins and capillaries. The function of the circulatory system is to transport oxygen, food, CO_2, and waste products to and from the cells of the body.

THE HEART

The heart is a muscular organ that pumps blood to the body and the lungs. It consists of four chambers, two collecting chambers (atria) and the pumping chambers (ventricles).

The Heart

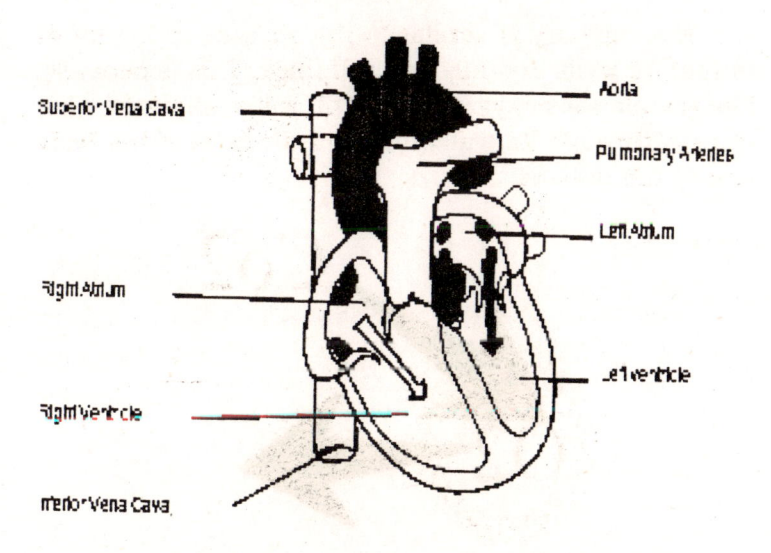

Fig. 9: The heart showing the flow of blood from the atria to the ventricles

THE BLOOD VESSELS

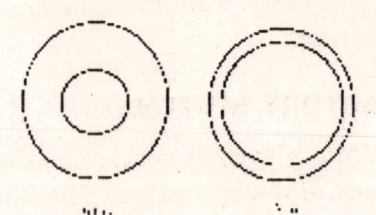

Fig. 10: Cross section of an artery and vein showing the difference in thickness

Both arteries and veins have three layers of tissue and in both the layers are a tough outer coat, a middle muscle layer and a smooth lining. The difference between the two is that the muscle layer is much thicker in the artery than in the vein. The artery requires a thick muscular wall so that it can assist in pumping blood around the body. The vein is soft so that blood can be squeezed along it by other muscles.

The capillary is similar to the air sacs in the lungs in that its walls are only one cell thick. This is because, like the air sacs oxygen and CO_2, water and food have to pass through its walls to get to the cells of the body and to the outside.

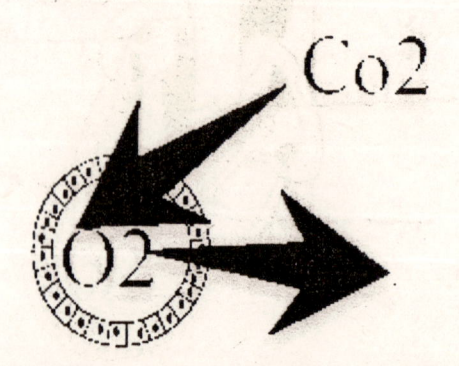

Fig. 11: Cross section of a capillary

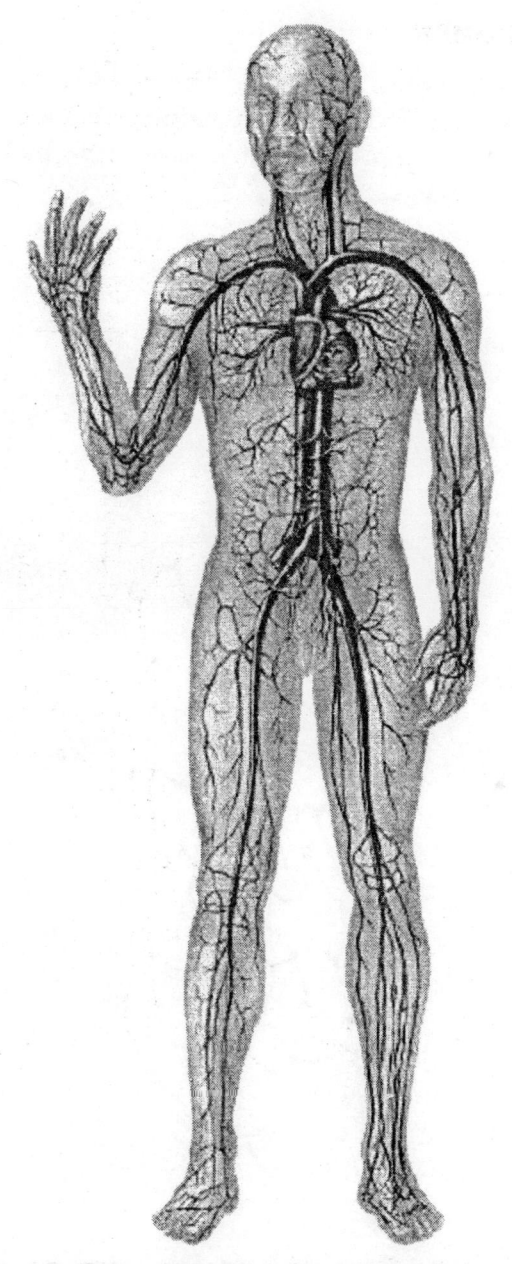

Fig. 12: The major blood vessels of the body

THE ABDOMEN

The abdomen contains the spleen, stomach, intestines, liver and pancreas, kidneys, bladder, female reproductive system and the blood vessels which supply them and the legs.

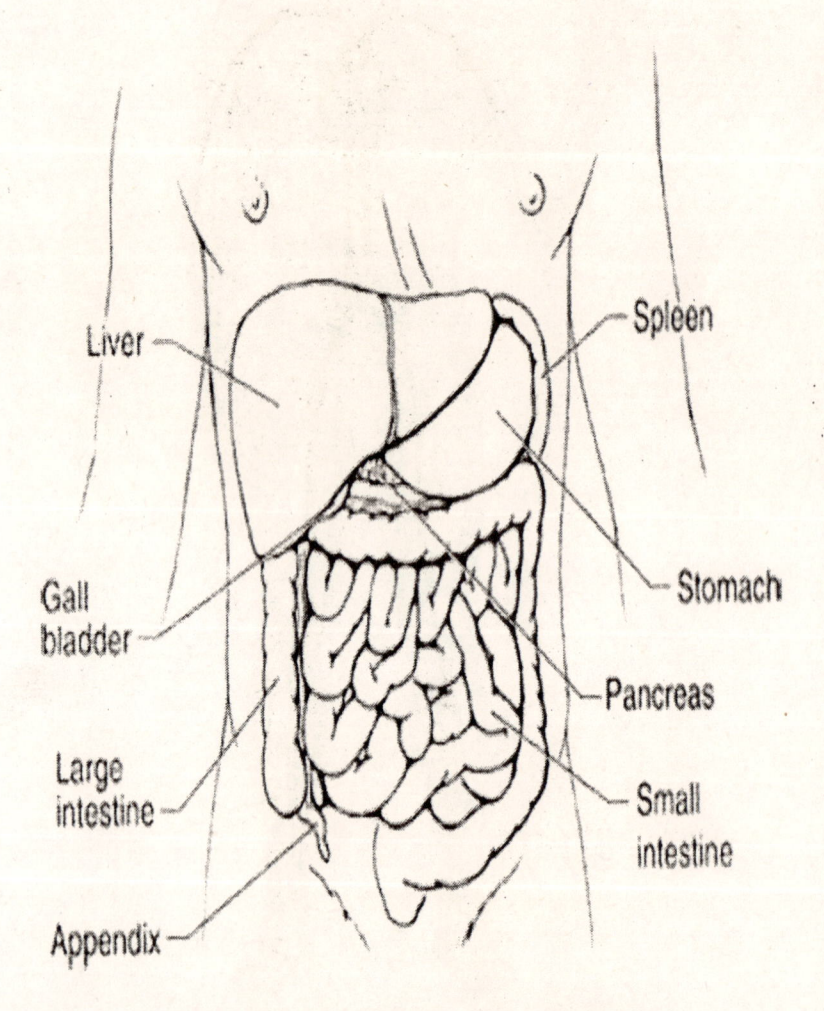

Fig. 13: The organs of the abdomen

THE SKIN

The skin comprises a number of layers and structures which protect the body from temperature change, damage, fluid loss and infection. What we see as skin is in fact the outermost layer which is dead.

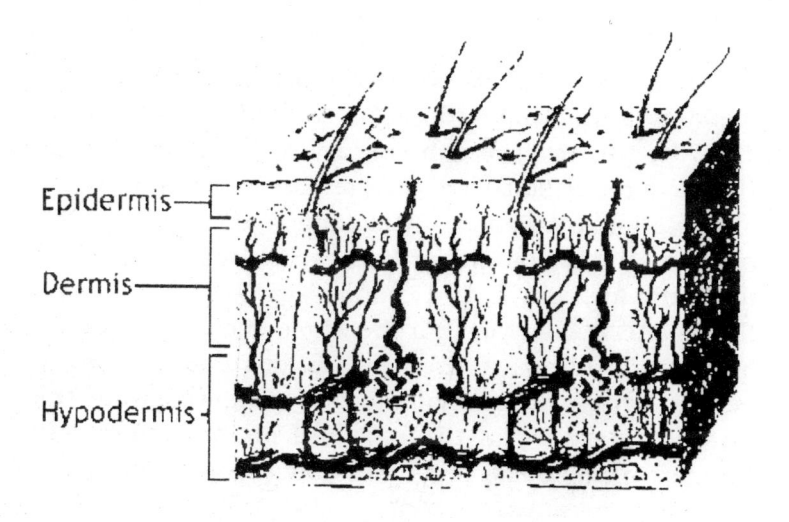

Fig. 14: Layers of the Skin

3

The Cells and Tissues

The word 'cell' derives from the Latin word cella, meaning a store or larder. The term was first used in 1665 by the seventeenth-century microscopist Robert Hooke to describe the spaces he observed in thin slices of cork. Hooke was actually looking at empty spaces left by cells, but the observation was important and led others to search for, and find, a cellular structure in all living things and to discover that the whole of biology is based on the cell. Although the cell has long been known to be the structural unit of the body, knowledge of the internal features of the cell and of the immensely complex biochemical processes going on in every living cell is comparatively recent.

The last fifty years or so has seen an explosive growth of knowledge of cell structure and function which has revolutionized medicine and is likely to have a greater effect on the future of mankind than any other branch of scientific advance. The body is made entirely of countless millions of cells and their products, and may be considered as a community of cells. Most of the cells are stuck together to form tissues but many, such as those in the blood, and those concerned with the immune system, are separate and free to move around.

Body cells vary greatly in size, from less than a hundredth of a millimetre across, in the case of red blood cells, with very long nerve fibres. The largest cell bodies are those of the egg, which is about a tenth of a millimetre across. Cells require fuel to provide them with energy,

The Cells and Tissues 35

and oxygen with which to burn up the fuel. Without such supplies they soon die. All cells are bathed in tissue fluid and supplies reach them by diffusion through this fluid.

The Cells Organs

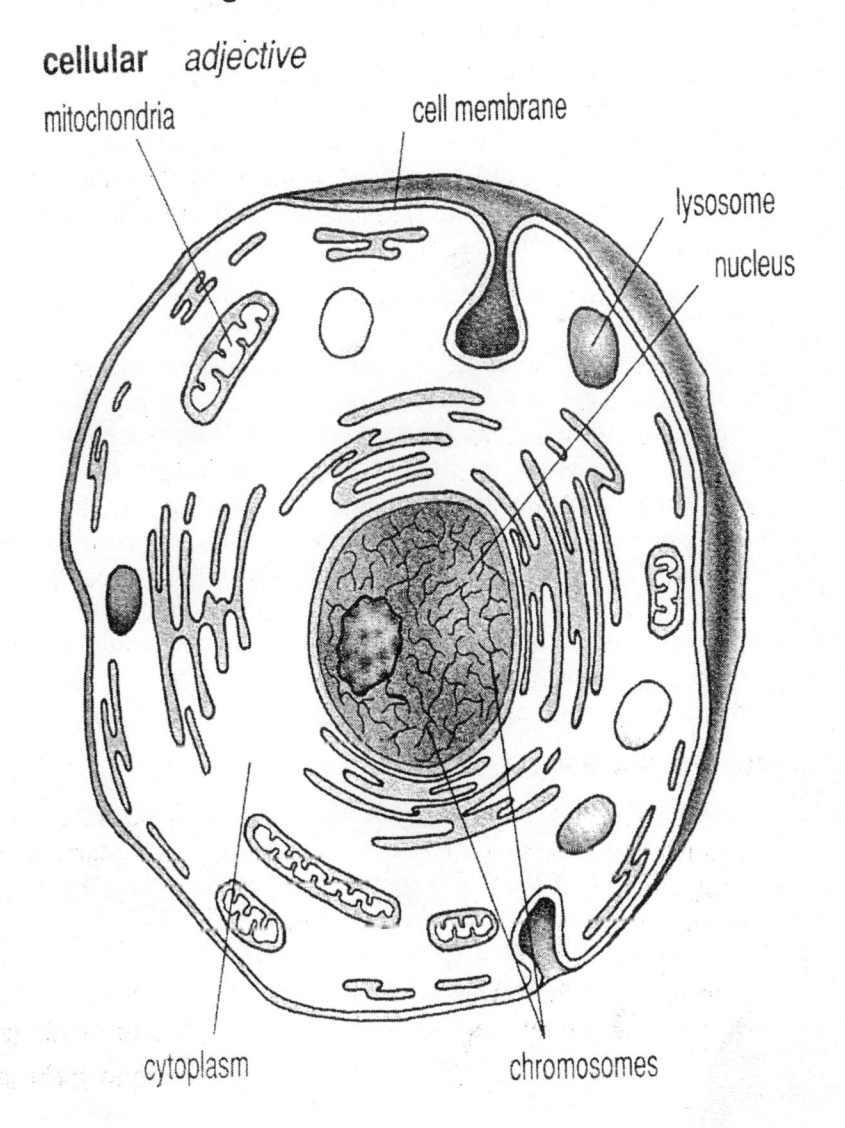

cellular *adjective*

mitochondria
cell membrane
lysosome
nucleus
cytoplasm
chromosomes

The cytoplasm also contains many important structures known as organelles or 'little organs'. Permeating the whole cytoplasm is the endoplasmic reticulum, a complex network of membrances, studded all over with tiny granules called ribosomes. These are dense collections of RNA and are the sites at which proteins are formed. Form the reticulum, newly made proteins are transported to other structures, known as the Golgi apparatus, named after the Italian histologist Camillo Golgi. The Golgi complexes are situated near the cell nucleus, and consist of a series of flattened, membranous sacs surrounded by a number of spherical bubbles, or vesicles.

These vesicles form initially on the surface of the rough reticulum in areas not coated with ribosomes. Proteins within the rough endoplasmic reticulum pass into these vesicles, which then travel though the cytoplasm and fuse on to the surface of the Golgi complex, transferring their contents into the Golgi sacs. Secondary transfer vesicles are now formed on the surface of the Golgi sacs, and these are 'tagged' by the addition of a carbohydrate or phosphate group to indicate where they should go. Golgi vesicles have been called the 'traffic police' of the cells as they play a key role in directing the many proteins that are formed within the cells to their required destination.

The Cell Nucleus

The central part of the cell which, in most stained sections under the microscope, appears much more densely coloured than the rest of the cell, is called the nucleus and contains the chromosomes—the coiled-up lengths of DNA that form the genetic blueprint for the reproduction of the cell and for the synthesis of proteins. Surrounding the nucleus, within the cell, is the fluid cytoplasm. Each cell type has a recognisable different cytoplasm, but in all cells this is mainly water, sometimes up to 97 per cent. Dissolved in the water are many substances such as proteins, including many enzymes, amino acids, nucleic acids, sugars, sodium, potassium, calcium, magnesium, iron, copper, zinc, iodine and bromine.

The mitochondria are thiny bags containing enzymes required for the building and breaking down processes of the cell and for the conversion of glucose and oxygen into energy. The are the power houses of the cell and contain rings of DNA of their own. This DNA is quite distinct from the DNA is the nucleus and is inherited only from the mother. Lyposomes are similar little sacs containing digestive enzymes capable of breaking down almost any organic molecule present in, or engulfed by, the cell. Lyposome enzymes act on materials taken in by cells in the process known as phagocytosis—literally 'cell eating'. They are especially conspicuous in the scavenging white cells of the immune system. The cell membranes are highly flexible structures made largely of a layer of fat molecules, mainly fats containing phosphorus held together by the basic forces that attract atoms to each other.

They also contain cholesterol, which is an essential constituent of every cell, and are penetrated by many large functional protein molecules. These cell membranes are far more than simple bags for the cell constituents. They are complex and important structures containing specialized protein sites for the receipt of information from the external environment and others for the pumping of dissolved chemical substances into and out of the cell. Our understanding of body function has been massively extended by the discovery that all cells possess such receptors, either on their surfaces, within their cytoplasm, or on the membranes surrounding their nuclei. Chemical messengers, such as hormones or neuro-transmitters are able to bind specifically to these receptors, and, in so doing, modify the function or actions of the cells. This, for instance, is how muscle cells are caused to contract and gland cells to secrete. Adrenaline receptors of three types occur on various cells and most have receptors for insulin. Many other hormones, prostaglandins and other chemical messengers bind to surface cell receptors. Steroids and the thyroid hormones enter cells and bind to receptors on the nuclei, prompting nuclear DNA to increase the transcription of particular genes.

Knowledge of the functioning of the brain has been greatly extended by advances in receptor site science, and this has also been very fruitful in the development of new drugs. Since the cell is so fundamental to

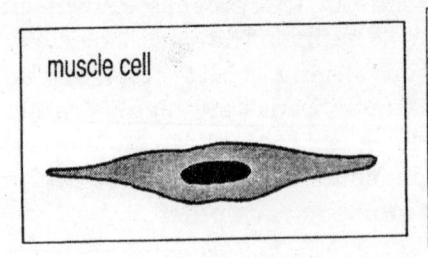

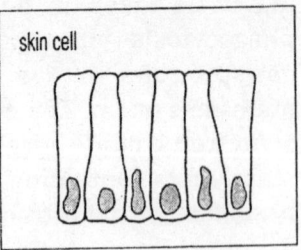

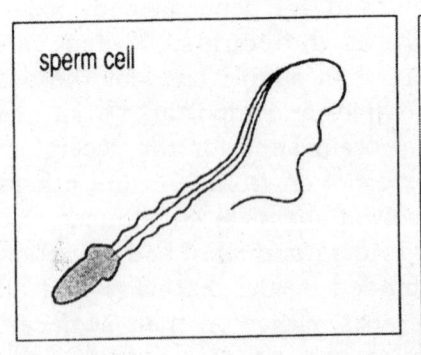

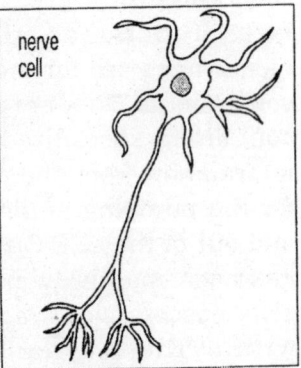

The Cells and Tissues.

medicine, this book necessarily contains a great deal more about cells, and especially about how cells can go wrong. Here, we are concerned only with the basic facts.

In the above shown figure, various kinds of cells present in human body have been represented. All these cells perform different kinds of functions which are very important for functioning of an human body properly.

COMPONENTS OF CELLS

There are many substances, which together made up the cells. Some of the important constituent of cells are as follows :—

a. Protoplasm : It is an important kind of matter which is being found in all kinds of cells. A large number of bio-molecules made up the protoplasms.

The essential anatomical features of the living cell may be described by reference to a generalized type of cell found in embryonic and adult connective tissue-commonly termed a fibroblast. Such a cell is composed

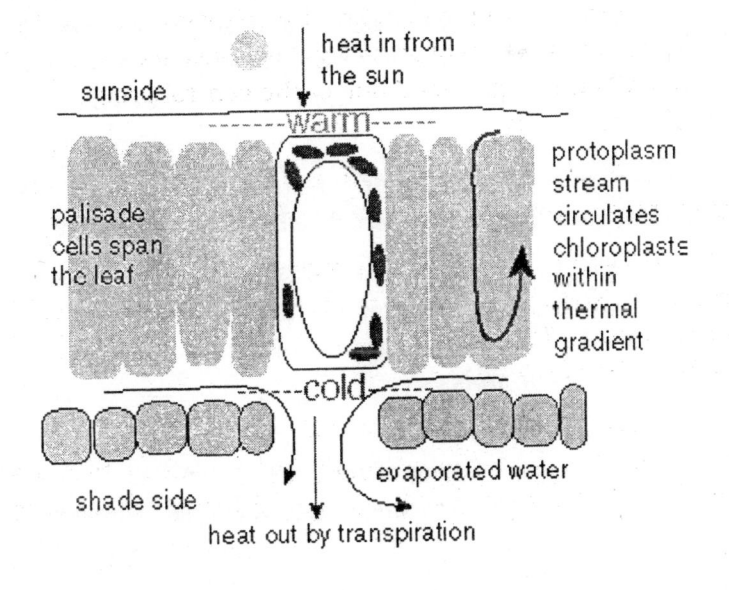

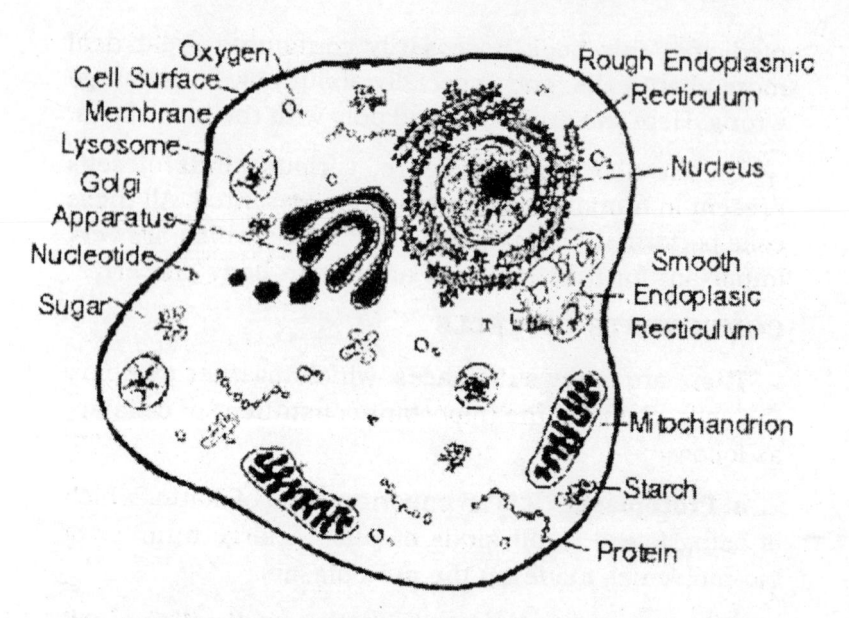

Diagram labels: Oxygen, Cell Surface Membrane, Lysosome, Golgi Apparatus, Nucleotide, Sugar, Rough Endoplasmic Recticulum, Nucleus, Smooth Endoplasic Recticulum, Mitochandrion, Starch, Protein

of a minute fragment of a jelly-like substance called protoplasm, in the middle of which is a rounded globule, the nucleus. The protoplasmic basis of the nucleus is termed the karyoplasm, and that of the cell body is which it is embedded, the cytoplasm. Since protoplasm is the material substratum of all living processes, its structural composition has provided one of the central problems of cytological study.

There are two different manner in which the protoplasm can be composed of, which are as follows :—

i. Inorganic : Elements like oxygen, hydrogen, carbon, nitrogen, sodium, potassium are the main constituents of this kind. They constitute around three to four per cent of the whole mass.

ii. Organic : Various kinds of compounds are being found in this type. Some of the important constituents are, fats, water, carbohydrate, water. All these substances enter into the human body through diet as they all are nutrient substances.

b. Cell Membranes : Different kinds of cells are being enclosed with the help of a thin covering, which is known as cell membrane. Outer boundary of the cell as well as its internal parts are being made up of cell membranes.

Cell membranes perform different kinds of functions, some of which are as follows :—

i. Internal or inner content of cell from out environment is being separated by the cell membrane.

ii. Various kinds of chemical messages are being received by this component and are being passed on to the cells.

iii. Cell's chemical reactions are being catalyzed by these membranes.

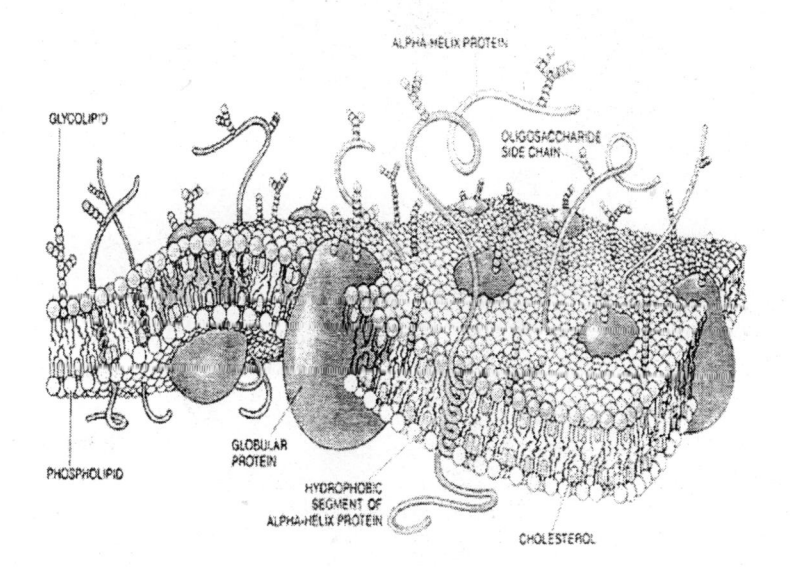

iv. Different types of molecules are being absorbed and excreted by these membranes.

c. Organelles : These are organisms which are small in size. A cell is made up of various little organs. Some of these organisms are covered with the help of thin covering, and some are without any kind of covering.

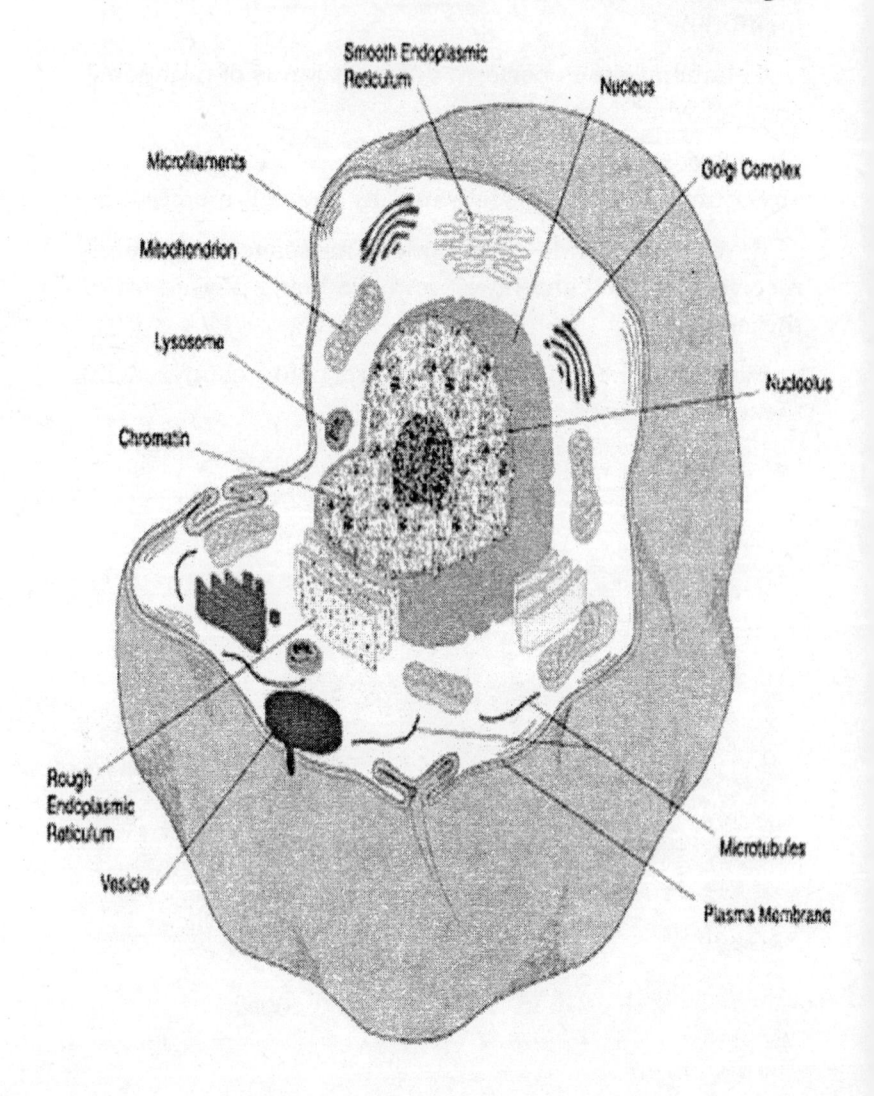

The Cells and Tissues 43

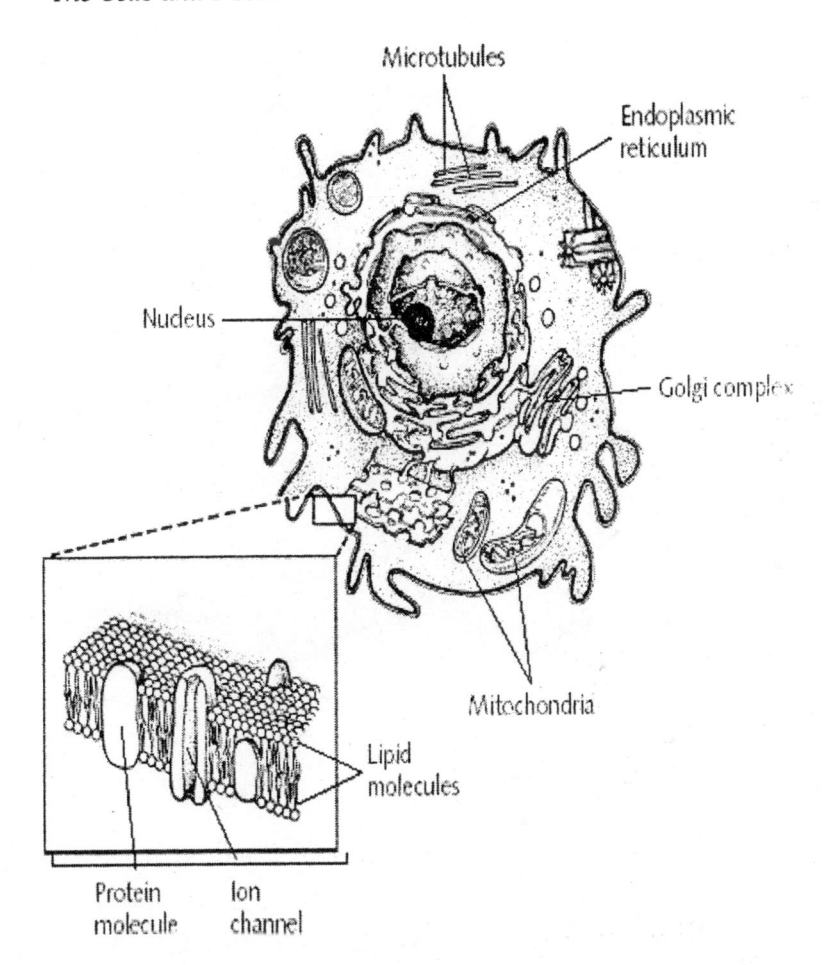

[Figure: Diagram of a cell with labels — Microtubules, Endoplasmic reticulum, Nucleus, Golgi complex, Mitochondria, Lipid molecules, Protein molecule, Ion channel]

d. Cytoplasm : The part of a cell between its membrane and nucleus is called the Cytoplasm. Between cell membrane and nuclue, there lies protoplasm. Within the cytoplasm of cells there are generally found certain essential elements called organelles which are now known to be of considerable functional significance, even though their function is not always clear. These include the mitochondria, the Golgi apparatus, and networks of flattened membranous sacs called endoplasmic reticula. All these structures are evidently important components of the living cell.

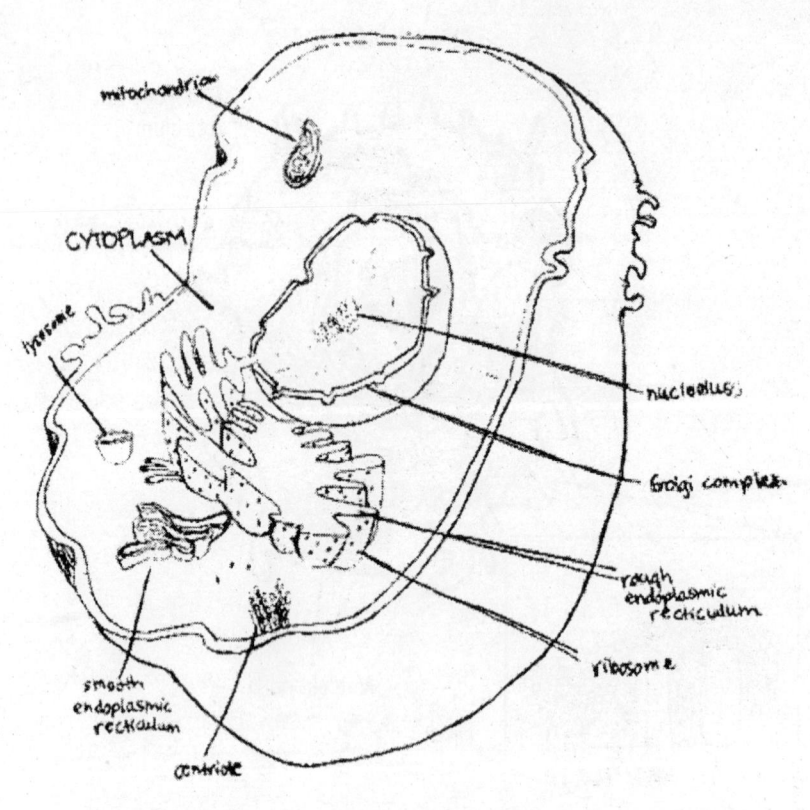

e. Mitochondria : Throughout the cytoplasm, small microscopic sacs are being found, which are called the Mitochondria. Outer smooth membrane and an inner membrane are main constituent of the mitochondria. Inner membrane is consisted of various folds, which consists of a number of enzymes. These enzymes perform different kinds of functions in human body.

Various important functions are being performed by Mitochondria, some of which are as follows :—

  i. There are important kind of enzymes in the

OUTER MEMBRANE

INNER MEMBRANE

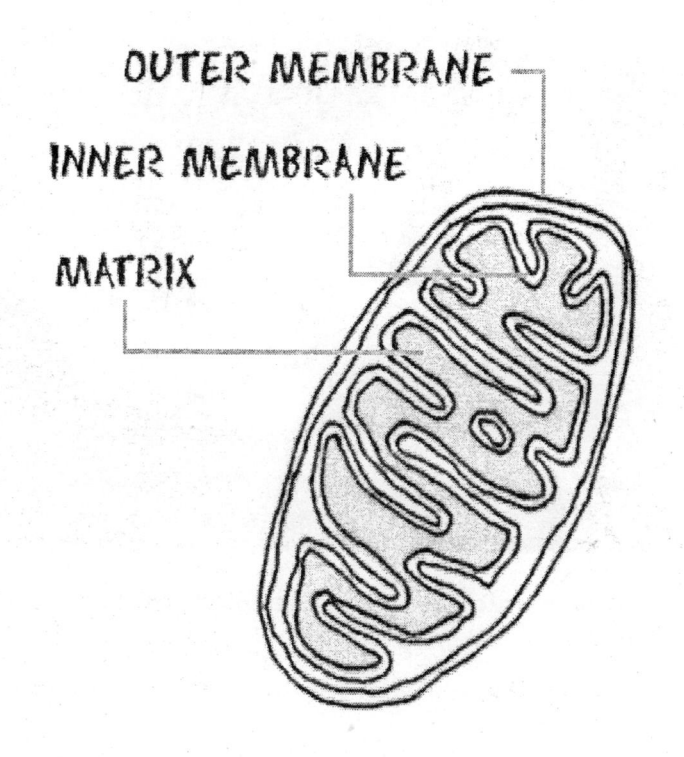

MATRIX

mitochondria, which perform different kinds of functions.

ii. They are considered or called the power house of the cell because they are main centre for production of energy.

iii. Adenosine Triphosephate is being transferred to the desired place in the human body by Mitochondria.

f. Lysosomes: These are the small membrane enclosed sacs, which consist of enzymes. These enzymes can break down various kinds of proteins and lipids.

Within the cell, lysosomes break down the large molecules. Digestion enzymes are being found in the

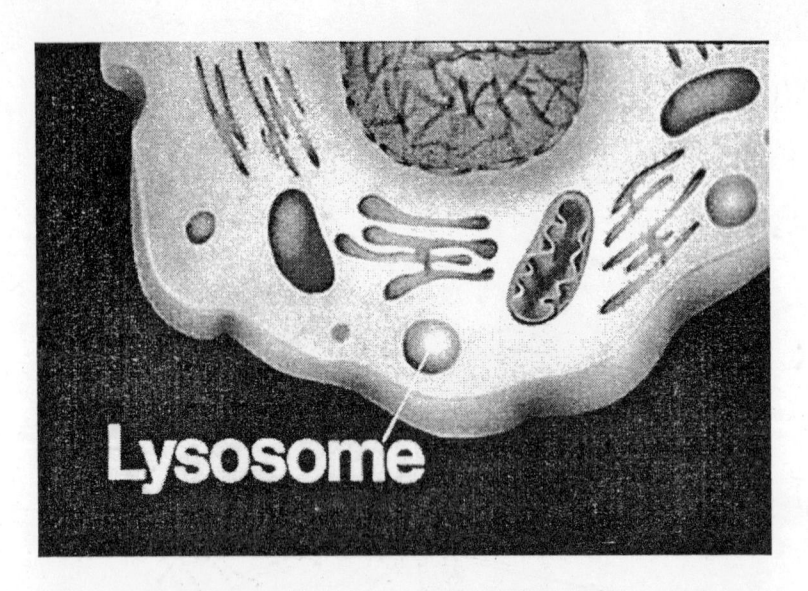

Lysosome

lysosomes, which help in digesting various kinds of food components.

g. Golgi Apparatus: The Golgi apparatus has been

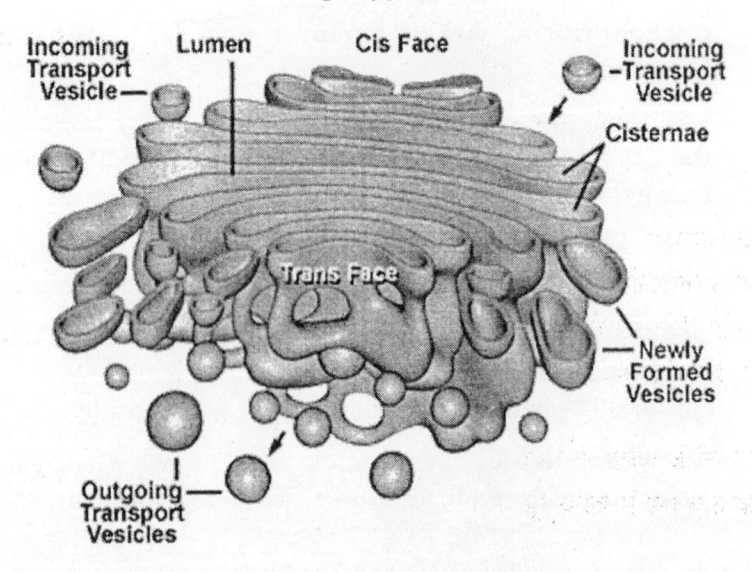

The Golgi Apparatus

The Cells and Tissues 47

described as a protoplasmic reticulum common to all types of cell. Usually situated around or in close proximity to the nucleus, it undergoes a characteristic displacement in glandular cells in relation of their secretory activity. In other cases it may become dispersed throughout the cytoplasm in the form of fine granules, and it undergoes rapid disintegration in degenerative conditions.

Golgi apparatus contains some special kind of enzymes, which perform the function of digestion. Movement of fluid in the cells and expulsion of recreatory products from the cells is being regulated by the golgi apparatus.

h. Ribosome: An individual cell is composed of number of ribosomes. These are the small spherical organs which remain attached to the endoplasmic reticulum and it is through the cytoplasm that they remain scattered.

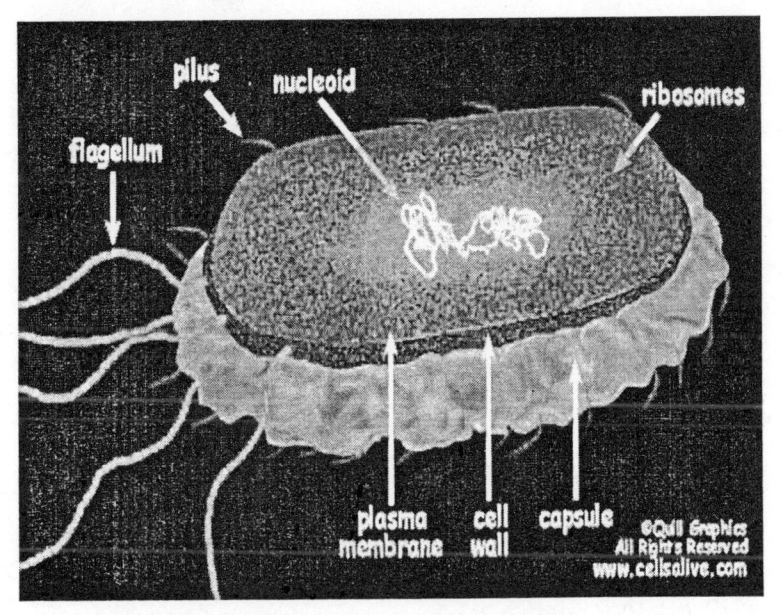

In the human body, protein component is being made up of ribosomes, and it is because of this reason that they are also called protection factors of the cells.

i. Vacuoles: These are sac like structures. These consist of water and water soluble substances. Various kinds of excretory functions are being done by this organ.

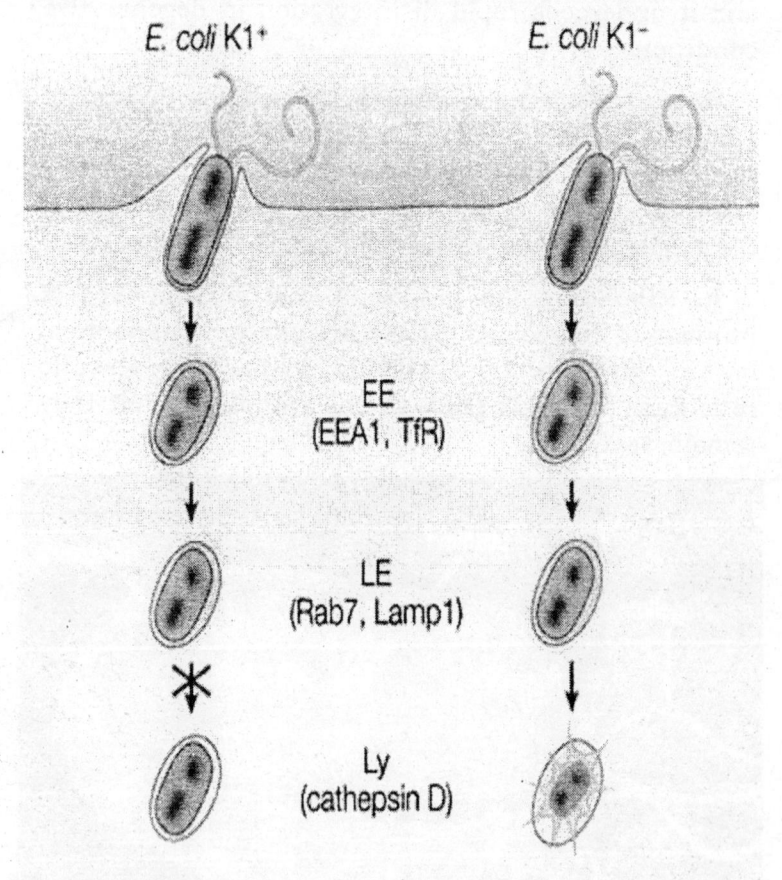

E. coli K1⁺   E. coli K1⁻

EE
(EEA1, TfR)

LE
(Rab7, Lamp1)

Ly
(cathepsin D)

Nature Reviews | Neuroscience

j. Cilia and Flagella: These are tiny hairs, the main purpose or function of which is to pull the cell through a fluid environment or to move the fluid surrounding the cell. Ciliar have a short length and they are being present in the human body in a great number. Generally, in the human respiratory tract, they are being found.

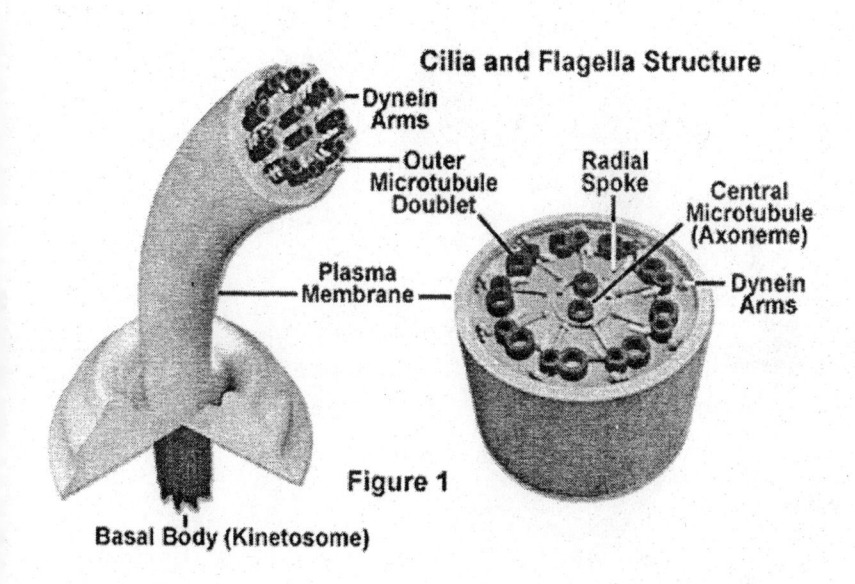

Cilia and Flagella Structure

Figure 1

Basal Body (Kinetosome)

k. Nucles: The nucleus of a generalized type of cell occupies an approximately central position in the cytoplasm, and it is enclosed in a definite membrane, the nuclear membrane. This is a double membrane and is not complete, for it may be interrupted at frequent intervals by small gaps, nuclear poses, that permit the transport of nuclear material into the surrounding cytoplasm, and of cytoplasmic material in the reverse direction. A nucleus usually contains one or two small, round and highly refractile particles, the nucleoli. In living cells, the nucleoli may show a rather irregular contour. Like the cytoplasm of the cell body, the karyoplasm of the nucleus appears in ordinary transmitted light to be a structurally homogeneous fluid in the normal living cell.

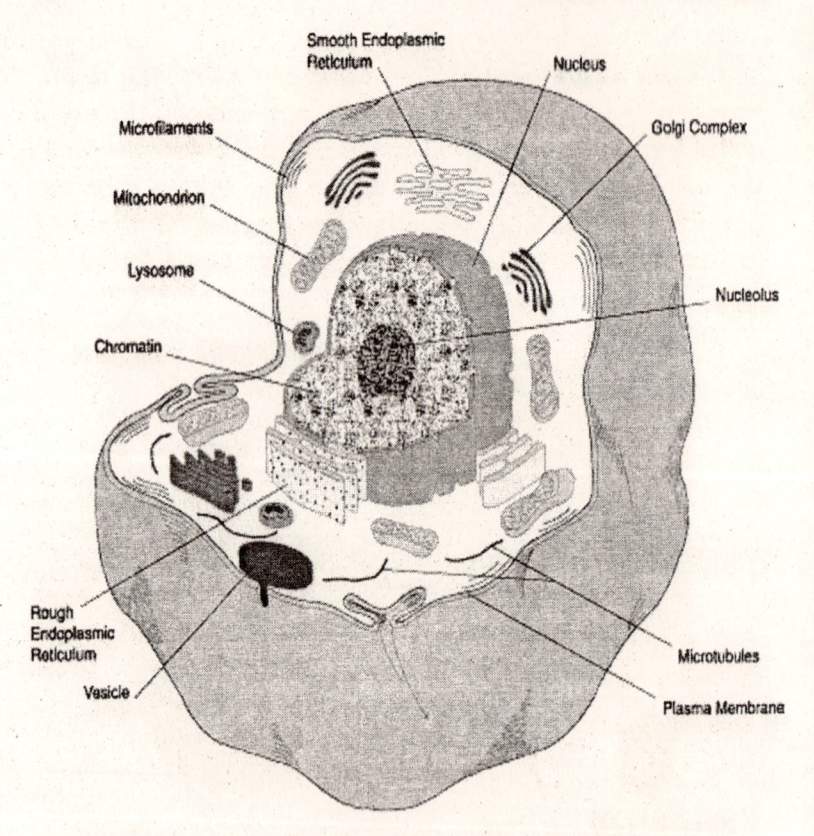

Nucleus control all cells in all the ways. The function of directing the cells growth and control of all the activities of the cell is being done by nucleoli. Various kinds of genetic information is also being controlled by nucleoli.

Two important kinds of structures that nucleus contains are nucleoli and chromosomes.

Nucleoli : These kinds of bodies can be found in specific places of chromosomes. Ribosome is being formed with the help of nucleoli. Proteins and Ribonucleic acids are the main constituents of nucleoli. In making proteins in the body, an important role is being played by Ribonucleic acid.

Chromosomes: These are long and very thin structures, which consists of certain proteins and Deoxyribo Nuclic Acid. Genes are made up of Deoxyribo Nuclic Acid, which are fundamental units of heredity.

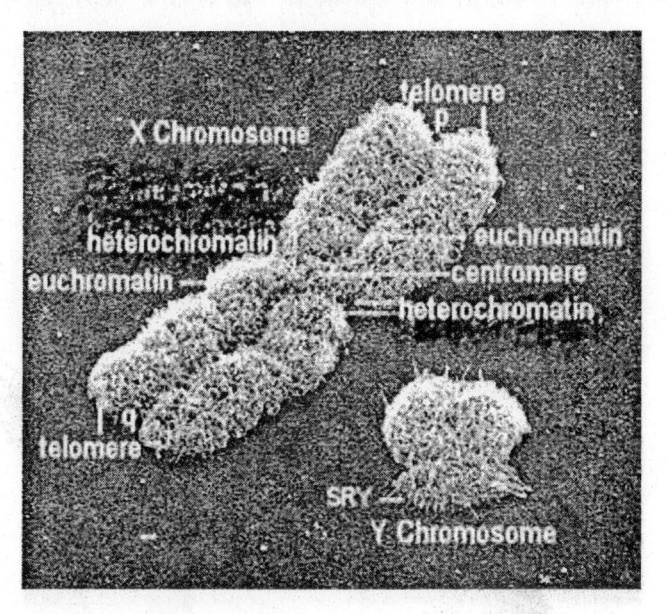

Process of Cell Division

At the time of origination, all the cells have a small size. It is after digestion process that it increases in the size. The limit to which it can grow it limited. After attaining a particular size, it gets divide into different parts to form new cells. This process of developing new cell with the result of division of old cell is known as cell division.

All cells which have not undergone extreme morphological specialization are normally capable of

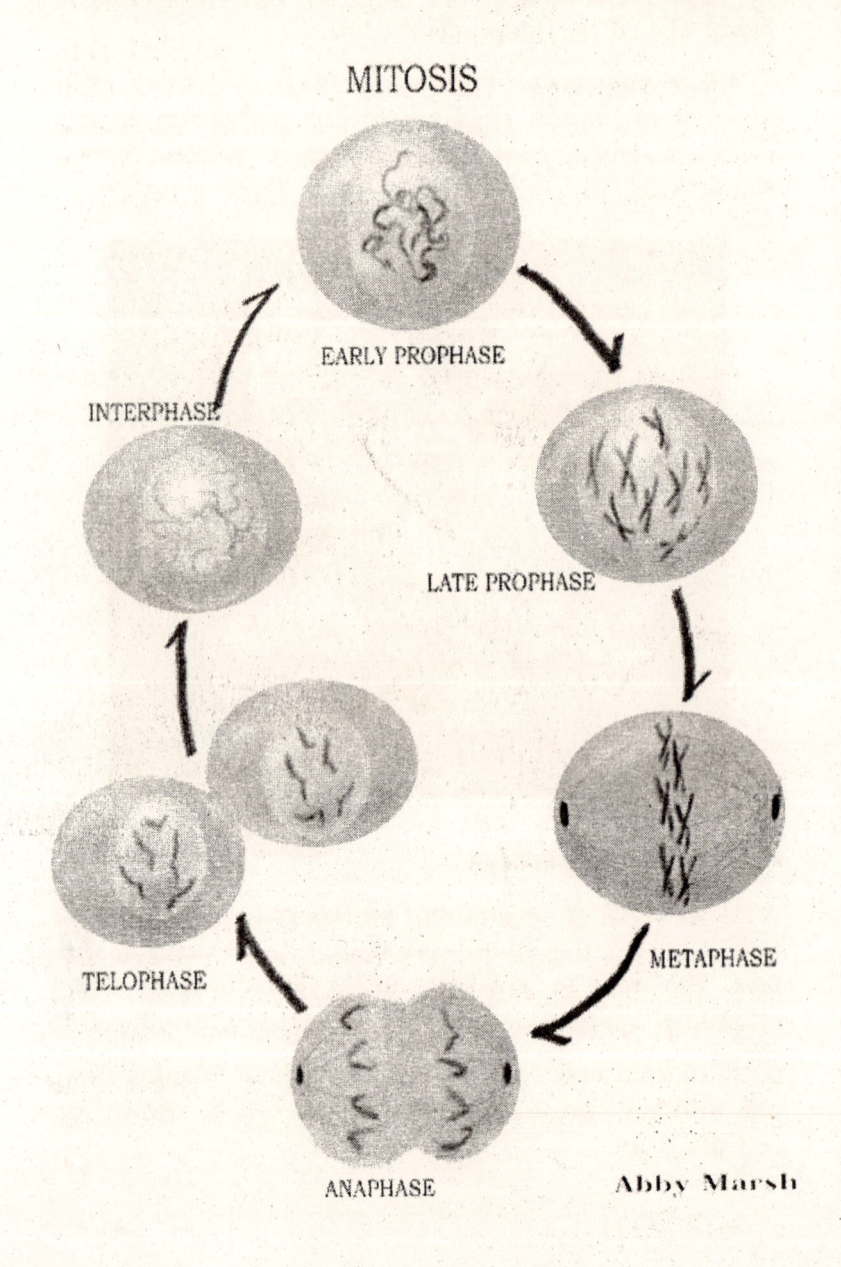

MITOSIS

EARLY PROPHASE

LATE PROPHASE

METAPHASE

ANAPHASE

TELOPHASE

INTERPHASE

Abby Marsh

The Cells and Tissues

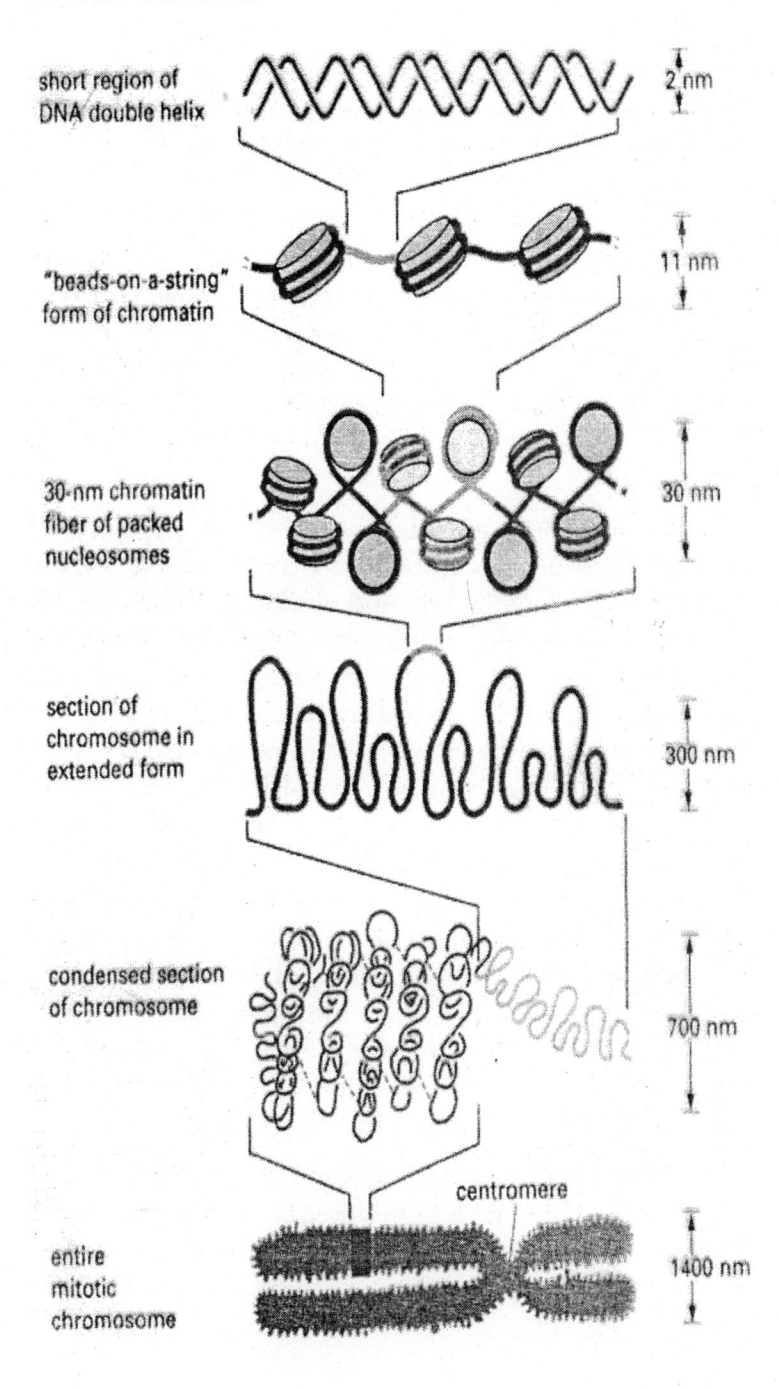

short region of DNA double helix	2 nm
"beads-on-a-string" form of chromatin	11 nm
30-nm chromatin fiber of packed nucleosomes	30 nm
section of chromosome in extended form	300 nm
condensed section of chromosome	700 nm
entire mitotic chromosome (centromere)	1400 nm

proliferation by dividing. The usual mechanism of cell division is the rather complicated process of mitosis, but the cells of some tissues have been stated to divide occasionally by the simpler method of amitosis, which involves a direct constriction and splitting of the nucleus without any apparent preliminary anatomical changes in the latter. It is now well established that true amitosis never does occur in normal ammalian tissue; such cases as were reported were evidently those in which an intranuclear rearrangement of chromatin remained undetected by the histological methods employed.

Thus, it is through the process of cell division that new cells give on originating in the body as from time to time, existing cells become dead and it becomes necessary to replace them with new cells. There are some cells in our body, which keeps in dividing throughout the life of an individual. All the cells are not of this nature. Some of the cells in our body cannot be replaced by new cells once they have died.

TISSUES

In organism, next level after cell is called tissue. Tissues are organised forms of cells. Various kind of special functions are being done by tissues, which serve the body as a whole. Tissues are made up of different kinds of cells. In various organs, there exists tissues in varying numbers, and each kind of tissue in an organ performs different kinds of functions.

In the muscular part of intestine, there exists a group of muscle cells, which make up or constitute the muscular tissue. Other kinds of cells are being present in the internal lining of the intestine. Muscular tissue

The Cells and Tissues

CELLS

↓

TISSUES

↓

ORGANS

↓

SYSTEMS

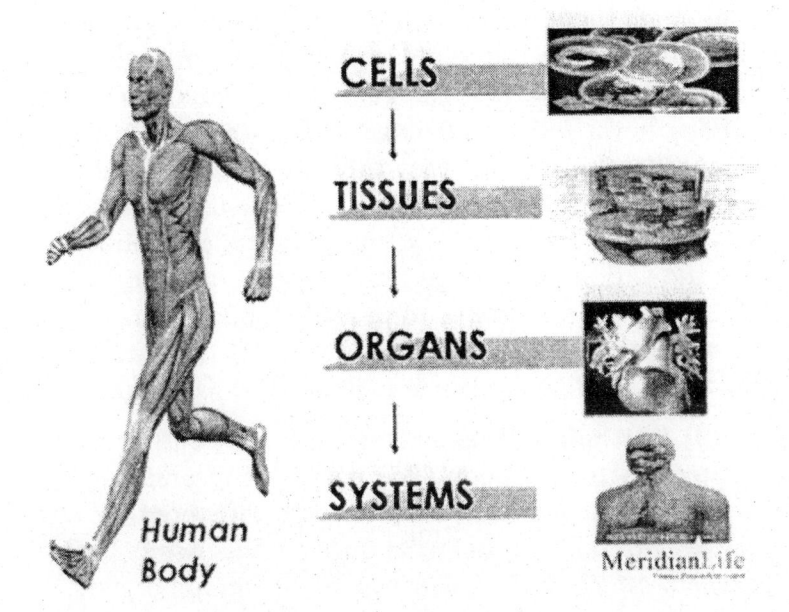

Human Body

MeridianLife

and lining tissues perform different kinds of functions. The function of muscular tissue to enable the food to move forward while the lining tissue performs the function of secreting the digestive juices while digesting the food. It is because of this reason that it is said that all the tissues present in human organs are of specialized nature.

Different kinds of tissues are being present in human being, some of the important are as follows :—

   a. Connective Tissue,

   b. Epithelial Tissue,

   c. Nervous Tissue, and

   d. Muscle Tissue.

(A) Connective Tissue: The skeleton keeps the organs, blood vessels and nerves in place and to a certain extent, provide some protection. The connective tissue supports and binds them together. It also supplies the ligaments and tendons for the joints and muscles, the tethering for the larger organs, the softness for protection and rigidity in the form of cartilage. There are many forms of connective tissue, but they are all developed from the same jelly-like ground substance, made up of salts and water, protein and carbohydrate. Embedded in this jelly are the various fibres and cells; elastic fibres to provide elasticity; collagen fibres to provide support; white cells and macrophages to fight infection; fat cells used for storage; and finally plasma cells to produce antibodies.

(B) Epithelial Tissue: This kind of tissue provides protection to the body. The whole body and various organs situated in the body are being covered by this tissue. Not only on the outer surface, this tissue is also present on the interior surface of the various organs.

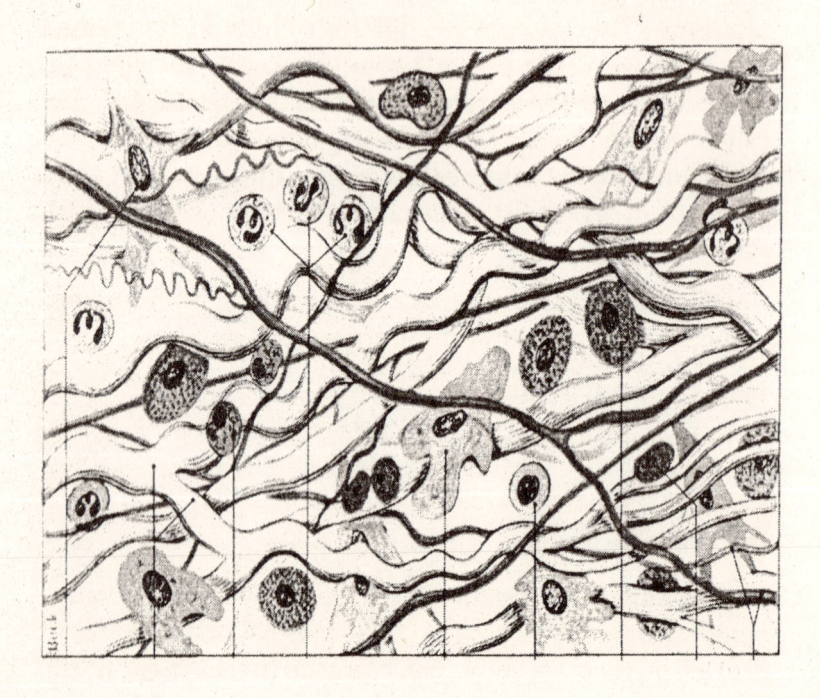

The shapes of these cells depend to a lot of extent on their function and the place where they locate in the body. They can have any shape. Individual cells situate very close to each other without any gap in between them and this feature makes these tissues the most ideal protective tissue.

(C) Nervous Tissue: Nerve cells or neurons are the main constituent of nervous tissues. Cell body is the main component of nerve cell. This nerve cell consists of nucleus and axon, which has a very long structure. There exist nerve fibres, which result because nerve cells are joined end to end. A nerve is composed of various nerve fibres. The message from one part of the body to another is being travelled through these nerves. Nervous tissues compose brain and spinal cord.

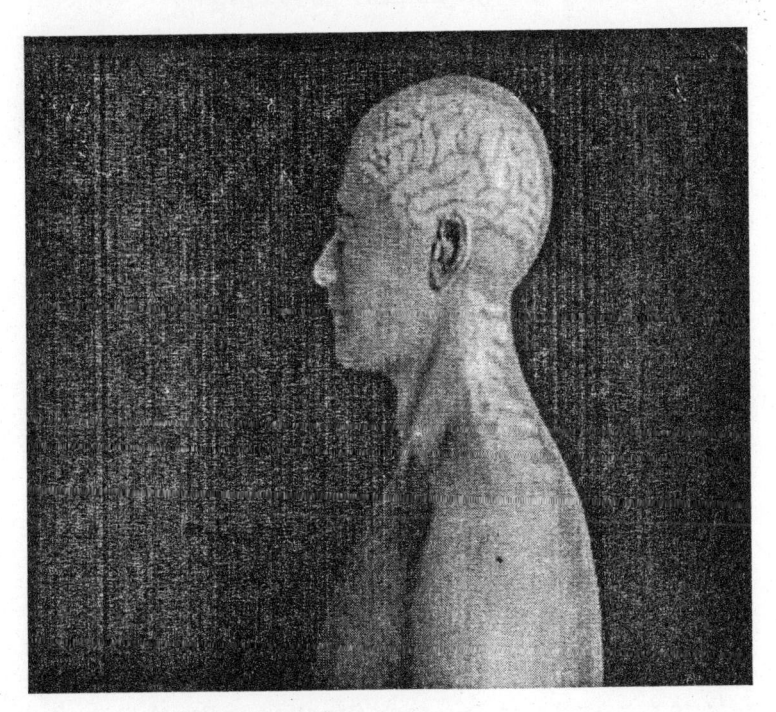

(D) Muscular Tissue: There exists a number of muscles in human body and these muscles are being formed by the muscular tissues. In every part of the body where movement is involved, muscular tissues are being found. It is considered to be the most important tissue of the body. More than one-third of the weight of the body is made up of muscular tissues.

Large number of muscles cells combine together to form the muscular tissue. With the help of connection tissue, muscle cells are being connected to each other. It is to the bones of the skeleton that most of the muscles are being attached. Such muscles can contract and expand, which help various parts of the body to move. Three different kinds of muscular tissues are present in the human body, which are as follows :—

a. Voluntary Muscles : Such kind of muscles are related to the bones of the human body and it is because of these muscles that they can move in some specific directions. These muscles cannot be moved without the will or efforts of the human beings, because of which they are being called the voluntary muscles.

In other words, those muscles which move only when we do some specific activities, are known as voluntary muscles.

b. Involuntary Muscles : As the name suggests, human beings do not have any control over these muscles. These muscles get moved on their own. Whether human beings want them to move or not, they get moved at their own will. In the walls of most internal body organs, such muscles are being present.

c. Heart Muscles : It is only in the heart that such kind of muscles are being found. These muscles have strong contractions and they function without stopping throughout the live. They are involuntary in nature.

THE NUCLEUS

The nucleus of a generalized type of cell occupies an approximately central position in the cytoplasm, and it is enclosed in a definite membrane, the nuclear membrane. This is a double membrane and is not complete, for it may be interrupted at frequent intervals by small gaps, nuclear poses, that permit the transport of nuclear material into the surrounding cytoplasm, and of cytoplasmic material in the reverse direction. A nucleus usually contains one or two small, round and highly refractile particles, the nucleoli. In living cells, the nucleoli may show a rather irregular contour. Like the cytoplasm of the cell body, the karyoplasm of the nucleus appears in ordinary transmitted light to be a structurally homogeneous fluid in the normal living cell.

In fixed and stained preparations, however, it show a fine network interspersed in which are minute granules. The substance of which the network is composed is commonly called chromatin, because it shows a marked affinity for basic dyes, and in its chemical composition it is characterized by its rich content of nucleoproteins. Phase-contrast microscopy has now demonstrated that the filaments and granules of the chromatin network visible in the stained nucleus actually exist as morphological entities in the living cell. They are invisible in unstained cells under the ordinary light microscope only because their refractive index is almost the same as that of the medium in which they are embedded.

However, the fact that, by micromanipulative methods, the nucleolus may be moved about quite easily within the nucleus has been taken to indicate that the filaments can hardly form a rigid meshwork, though of course, these methods are perhaps open to the criticism that they may effect rapid liquefactive changes in the normal constitution of the chromatin of the undamaged nucleus by mechanical injury. Of considerable interest is the recent discovery that a sex difference can be recognized in the chromatin content of the nuclei of many types of somatic cell, for in the female of some mammals a special chromatin mass, the sex chromatin, is usually to be seen as a small compact body in close contact with the nuclear membrane or as a little satellite related to the nucleolus. A similar structure is only rarely to be detected in the nucleus of males.

In typical cells there is but one nucleus, but in some there are two or more. This may be the result of the incomplete separation of cells after division, or the fusion of originally separate cells.

CELL INCLUSION

Within the cytoplasm are frequently to be found particles of inert, non-living material which are either taken up secondarily by the cell from the surrounding medium or else are products of its own activity. They are to be distinguished from the organized living contents of cytoplasm which have already been described and which are termed organelles. In the case of cells which are actively motile or amoeboid, the cytoplasm may contain a variety of ingested material as, for instance, the remains of cell debris removed in the process of repair after tissue destruction or foreign particles such as bacteria.

4

Bones, Joints and Skeletal System

BONES

Bone is the important part of human body. Our entire body's framework are made up of different kinds of body. There are 206 bones existed in our body. Our Skeletal System provides support to delicate inner organs like liver, heart, kidney, intestines etc., that plays an important role in the functioning of human body. Bone is mostly made up of calcium slats, held together with strong fibres. It is usually hollow, and bone marrow and minerals are stored inside. There are two kinds of bone. Compact bone is hard and solid. Cancellous bone looks spongy. Humans have about 200 long and short bones.

Bones are rigid organs that form part of the endoskeleton of vertebrates. They function to move, support, and protect the various organs of the body, produce red and white blood cells and store minerals. Bone tissue is a type of dense connective tissue. Because bones come in a variety of shapes and have a complex internal and external structure they are lightweight, yet strong and hard, in addition to fulfilling their many other functions. One of the types of tissue that makes up bone is the mineralized osseous tissue, also called bone tissue, that gives it rigidity and a honeycomb-like three-dimensional internal structure. Other types of tissue found in bones include marrow, endosteum and periosteum, nerves, blood vessels and cartilage. There are 206 bones in the adult human body and 270 in an infant.

Functions: Bones have ten main functions:

Mechanical

• ***Protection*** — Bones can serve to protect internal organs, such as the skull protecting the brain or the ribs protecting the heart and lungs.

• ***Shape*** — Bones provide a frame to keep the body supported.

• ***Movement*** — Bones, skeletal muscles, tendons, ligaments and joints function together to generate and transfer forces so that individual body parts or the whole body can be manipulated in three-dimensional space. The interaction between bone and muscle is studied in biomechanics.

• ***Sound transduction*** — Bones are important in the mechanical aspect of overshadowed hearing.

Synthetic

• ***Blood production*** — The marrow, located within the medullary cavity of long bones and interstices of cancellous bone, produces blood cells in a process called haematopoiesis.

Metabolic

• ***Mineral storage*** — Bones act as reserves of minerals important for the body, most notably calcium and phosphorus.

• ***Growth factor storage*** — Mineralized bone matrix stores important growth factors such as insulin-like growth factors, transforming growth factor, bone morphogenetic proteins and others.

• **Fat Storage**— The yellow bone marrow acts as a storage reserve of fatty acids

• **Acid-base balance**— Bone buffers the blood against excessive pH changes by absorbing or releasing alkaline salts.

• **Detoxification**— Bone tissues can also store heavy metals and other foreign elements, removing them from the blood and reducing their effects on other tissues. These can later be gradually released for excretion.[citation needed]

• **Endocrine organ**— Bone controls phosphate metabolism by releasing fibroblast growth factor - 23, which acts on kidney to reduce phosphate reabsorption.

Individual Bone Structure

A femur with a cortex of compact bone and medulla of trabecular boneBone is not a uniformly solid material, but rather has some spaces between its hard elements.

Compact bone or (Cortical bone)

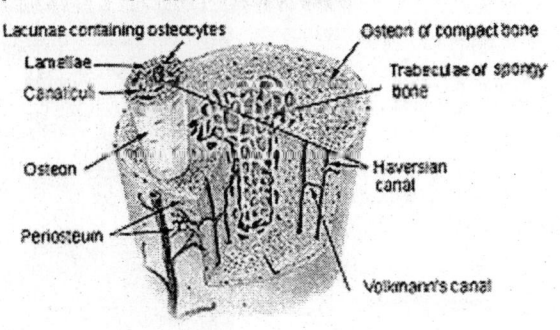

The hard outer layer of bones is composed of compact bone tissue, so-called due to its minimal gaps and spaces. This tissue gives bones their smooth, white, and solid appearance, and accounts for 80% of the total bone mass of an adult skeleton. Compact bone may also be referred to as dense bone.

Trabecular Bone

Filling the interior of the organ is the trabecular bone tissue (an open cell porous network also called cancellous or spongy bone), which is composed of a network of rod- and plate-like elements that make the overall organ lighter and allowing room for blood vessels and marrow. Trabecular bone accounts for the remaining 20% of total bone mass but has nearly ten times the surface area of compact bone.

Cellular Structure

There are several types of cells constituting the bone;

Osteoblasts are mononucleate bone-forming cells that descend from osteoprogenitor cells. They are located on the surface of osteoid seams and make a protein mixture known as osteoid, which mineralizes to become bone. Osteoid is primarily composed of Type I collagen. Osteoblasts also manufacture hormones, such as prostaglandins, to act on the bone itself. They robustly produce alkaline phosphatase, an enzyme that has a role in the mineralisation of bone, as well as many matrix proteins. Osteoblasts are the immature bone cells.

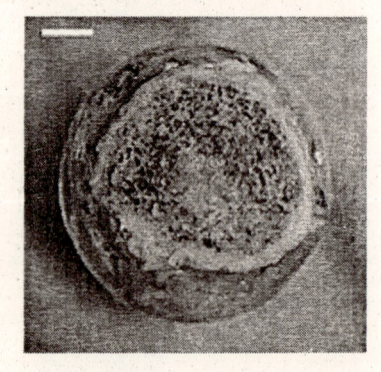

Bone lining cells are essentially inactive osteoblasts. They cover all of the available bone surface and function as a barrier for certain ions.

Osteocytes originate from osteoblasts that have migrated into and become trapped and surrounded by bone matrix that they themselves produce. The spaces they occupy are known as lacunae. Osteocytes have many processes that reach out to meet osteoblasts and other osteocytes probably for the purposes of communication. Their functions include to varying degrees: formation of bone, matrix maintenance and calcium homeostasis. They have also been shown to act as mechano-sensory receptors—regulating the bone's response to stress and mechanical load. They are mature bone cells.

Osteoclasts are the cells responsible for bone resorption (remodeling of bone to reduce its volume). Osteoclasts are large, multinucleated cells located on bone surfaces in what are called Howship's lacunae or resorption pits. These lacunae, or resorption pits, are left behind after the breakdown of the bone surface. Because the osteoclasts are derived from a monocyte stem-cell lineage, they are equipped with phagocytic like mechanisms similar to circulating macrophages. Osteoclasts mature and/or migrate to discrete bone surfaces. Upon arrival, active enzymes, such as tartrate resistant acid phosphatase, are secreted against the mineral substrate.

THE JOINTS

Joints are junctions between bones, and the term is applied whether or not obvious movement is possible. There are three types of joints—fibrous, cartilagineous and synovial, all of which have been shown with diagram below:

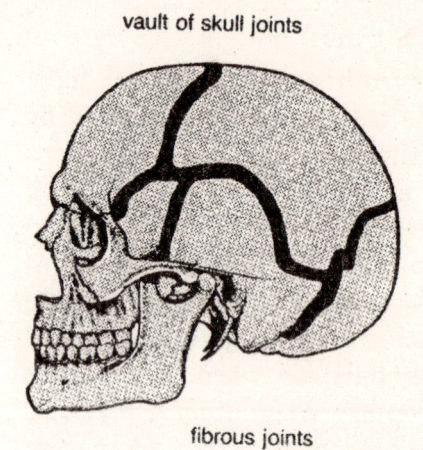

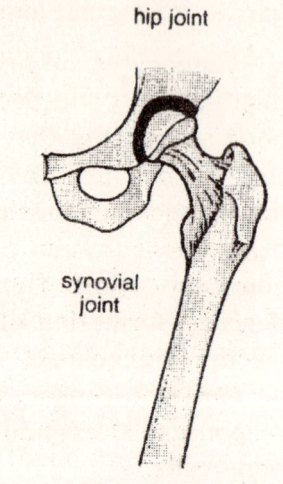

vault of skull joints

hip joint

synovial joint

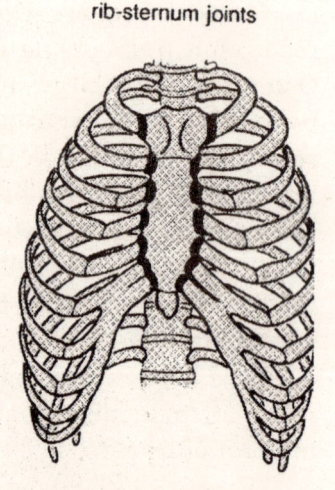

fibrous joints

rib-sternum joints

In fibrous joints, such as those between the spines of the vertebral column, the bones of the pelvis or the bones making up the skull, little or no movement is possible because the bones are held firmly together by ligaments. Cartilagineous joints, such as those between the ribs and the breast bone, have flexible cartilage fusing the bones together, allowing some limited movement. Synovial joints, are freely movable. Although the bearing surfaces of synovial joints are covered with cartilage, there is a space between these surfaces which is well lubricated with a fluid known as synovial fluid. The whole joint is enclosed in a capsule of tough fibrous tissue lined with the synovial membrane, which secretes synovial fluid.

Synovial joints may be:

1. Rotating joints, as in the head of the radius at the elbow, and between the upper two vertebrae of the spine;

2. 'Ball-and-socket' joints, as in the shoulder and hip, allowing some movement in any direction:

3. Sliding joints, as at the wrists and in the feet. Some sliding also occurs at the knee joints.

4. Hinge joints, as in the fingers and knees, allowing movement in one plane only.

In all cases, the range of possible movement is restricted by ligaments, which may be external to the joint, internal, or both.

THE SKELETAL SYSTEM

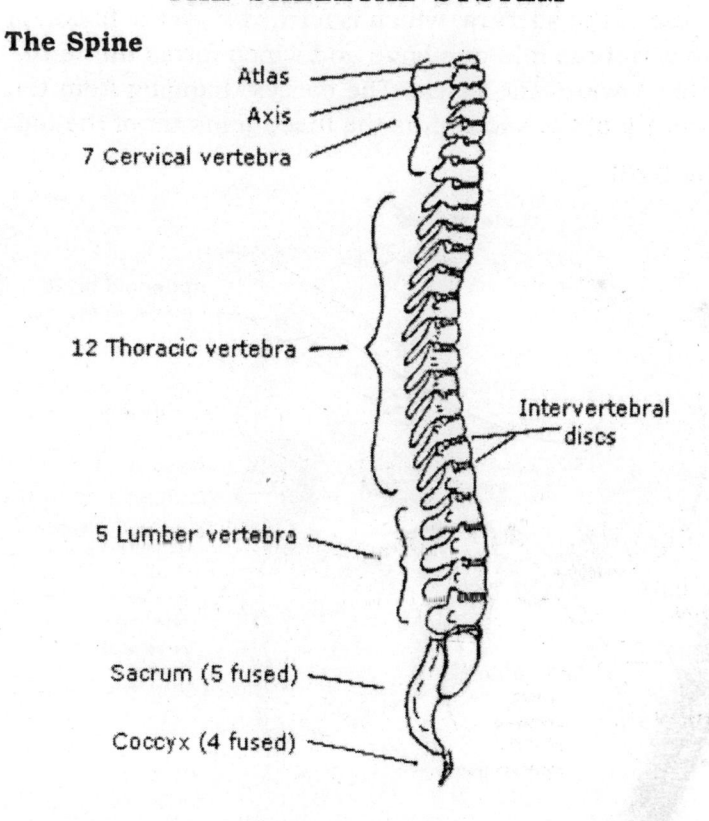

The Spine

- Atlas
- Axis
- 7 Cervical vertebra
- 12 Thoracic vertebra
- Intervertebral discs
- 5 Lumber vertebra
- Sacrum (5 fused)
- Coccyx (4 fused)

The spine, or vertebral column, is a curved column of individual bones, called vertebrae, all of the same general shape but varying progressively in size and proportion from the top of the column to the bottom. Each vertebra consists of a stout, roughly circular body in front, and an arch behind, enclosing an opening to accommodate the spinal cord. The bones fit neatly together, the bodies being separated by the intervertebral disc and the arches making contact by four smooth surfaces, two above and two below. The vertebrae in the neck are the smallest but have the largest cord opening.

Those at the bottom of the column are massive. There are seven vertebrae for the neck, twelve for the back and five for the lumbar region. The fifth lumbar vertebra sits on top of the sacrum, which is formed from the fusion of five vertebrae into one bone and which forms the centre of the back of the pelvis. The coccyx, hanging from the lower tip of the sacrum, is the fused remnant of the tail.

The Skull

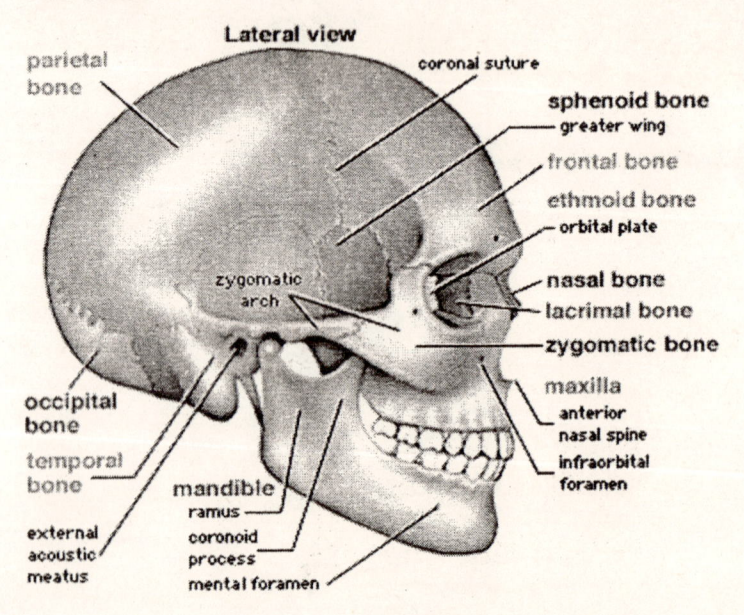

Lateral view

- parietal bone
- coronal suture
- sphenoid bone
  - greater wing
- frontal bone
- ethmoid bone
  - orbital plate
- zygomatic arch
- nasal bone
- lacrimal bone
- zygomatic bone
- maxilla
  - anterior nasal spine
  - infraorbital foramen
- occipital bone
- temporal bone
- external acoustic meatus
- mandible
  - ramus
  - coronoid process
  - mental foramen

Frontal view

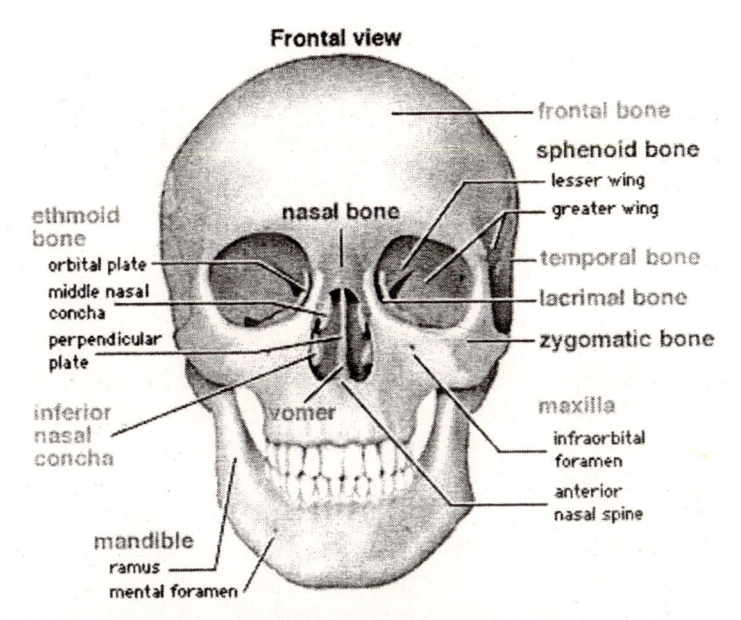

- frontal bone
- sphenoid bone
  - lesser wing
  - greater wing
- nasal bone
- temporal bone
- ethmoid bone
  - orbital plate
  - middle nasal concha
  - perpendicular plate
- lacrimal bone
- zygomatic bone
- inferior nasal concha
- vomer
- maxilla
  - infraorbital foramen
  - anterior nasal spine
- mandible
  - ramus
  - mental foramen

The brain, as the most important organ in the body, is correspondingly well protected and is entirely enclosed in, and supported by, the hollow skull. The interior of the skull is fashioned to fit precisely to the shape of the brain and contains three descending shelves to support the frontal lobes, the middle part of the brain, and the rear lobes and the hind brain. In the centre of the middle shelf is a hollow to accommodate the pituitary gland, and in the centre of the deep rear shelf is a large opening, the foremen magnum, through which the downward continuation of the brain, the spinal cord, passes into the canal of the spine. In the centre of the upper shelf, on either side of the midline, are two thin perforated bony plates through which the many fibres of the nerves of smell pass down into the nose.

Lying immediately under the outer parts of the front shelf are the two bony sockets which accommodate and protect the eyes. At the back of the orbits are holes in the bone to allow the optic nerves to pass back to the brain and to allow the nerves which move the eye muscles to run forward from the brain. To the inner side of each orbit, and separated from them by paper-thin sheets of bone, are separated from them by paper-thin sheets of bone, are two sets of sinuses, or air cells, the ethmoidal sinuses. The back wall of the nose is formed by the front of the bone forming the central shelf of the skull.

This bone is hollow and contains one or two sinuses. The pituitary gland is accessible, surgically, from the nose, through this wall. The floor of the nose is formed by the bony palate is a plate of bone which from part of the upper jaw. It is transversely ridged in young people but smooth in the old. The back edge of the hard palate is easily felt, in the mouth, and has a small protruding bump at each side. Under the orbits are the paired maxillary bones of the upper jaw. Like the sphenoid, these are hollow. They contain the maxillary sinuses, or antrums, and bear the upper teeth.

The hinged lower jaw carries a corresponding set of lower teeth. The jaw joins with the base of the skull at hinge joints high up in front of each ear. The heads of the mandible can be seen bulging the skin, just in front of the ears, when the mouth is opened widely. The mandible is pulled upwards by wide powerful muscles running down to it from the base of the skull and the outside of the temple bones. The latter can be felt to contract, on either side of the forehead, when the teeth are clenched. The vault of the skull consists of the wide forehead bone containing the frontal sinuses—air spaces between the two layers of hard bone of which the vault of the skull is made; the paired, upper and rear side bones; the paired lower front temporal bones; and the single lower rear occipital bone.

Infants have a gap, called a fontanelle, between the

upper parts of these bones. The prominence of the cheeks and part of the outer walls and floors of the orbits are formed by the zygomatic bones. The prominent bony process, which may be felt behind the lower part of the ear, is called the mastoid process. This is honeycombed with air cells and these communicate with the middle ear.

The Pelvic Girdle and Leg

The pelvis is the bony girdle formed by the junction of the two hip bones, on either side, with the triangular curved sacrum, behind, at the sacroiliac joints. The innominate bones are held together in front by a midline joint called thesymphysis pubis. Each innominate bone contains a deep, spherical cup, called the acetabulum, into which the head of the thigh bone fits. The sacroiliac joints are the semi-rigid ligamentous junctions, at the back, holding the two outer bones of the pelvis to the side surfaces of the sacrum.

The coccyx, or tail bone, consists of four small vertebrae fused together and joined to the curved sacrum. Normally little movement occurs at the curved sacrum. Normally little movement occurs at the sacroiliac joints, but late in pregnancy the strong ligaments holding the joints together become a little lax, to allow easier childbirth. The width of the hips is determined by the width of the pelvis and by the angle at which the heads of the two femurs joint it. The thigh bones are the longest and shortest bones in the body. Each has an almost spherical head which fits into a cup on the side of the pelvis. To the bottom end of each femur, at the knee, is attached the two lower leg bones, the stout tibia and the slender fibula—corresponding to the two bones of the forearm. The bottom ends of these bones joint the eight tarsal bones—corresponding roughly to the eight wrist bones, then the five metatarsal bones and the fourteen phalanges of the foot and toes. The big toe has two phalanges; the others three.

The Ribs

In the chest area, the vertebrae of the spinal column provide attachment for the twelve pairs of ribs, and most of these connect to the breast bone in front, thus forming the chest bony wall. The articulation of the ribs with the spine behind, and the breast bone in front, their shape, and the way each is suspended by a muscle from the one above, results in a considerable increase in the internal volume of the rib cage when the muscles between the ribs contract. The upper seven pairs of ribs are attached by flexible cartilages to the sternum.

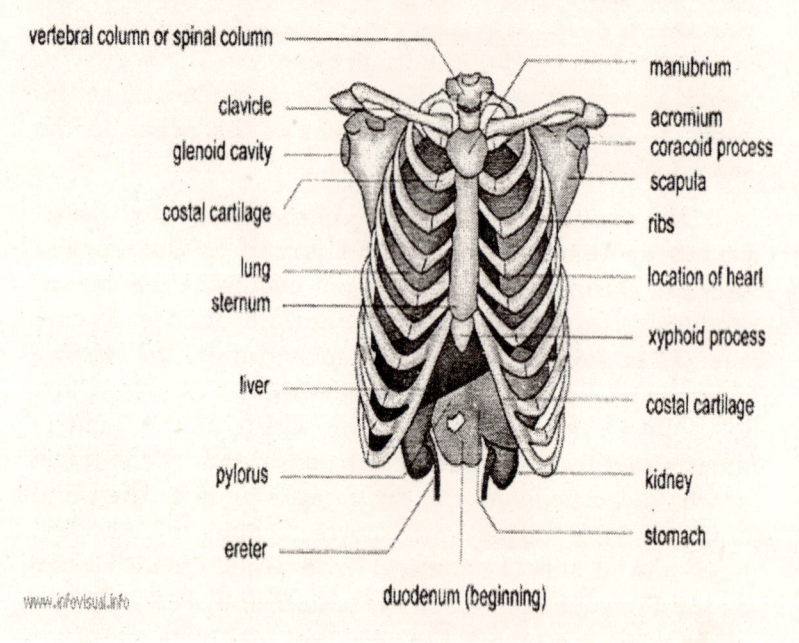

- vertebral column or spinal column
- clavicle
- glenoid cavity
- costal cartilage
- lung
- sternum
- liver
- pylorus
- ereter
- duodenum (beginning)
- manubrium
- acromium
- coracoid process
- scapula
- ribs
- location of heart
- xyphoid process
- costal cartilage
- kidney
- stomach

www.infovisual.info

The next three pairs, known as false ribs, are each connected by cartilage to the pair of ribs above. And the last two pairs, known as the floating ribs, are shorter and are not attached at the front. Occasionally, there is

Bones, Joints and Skeletal System

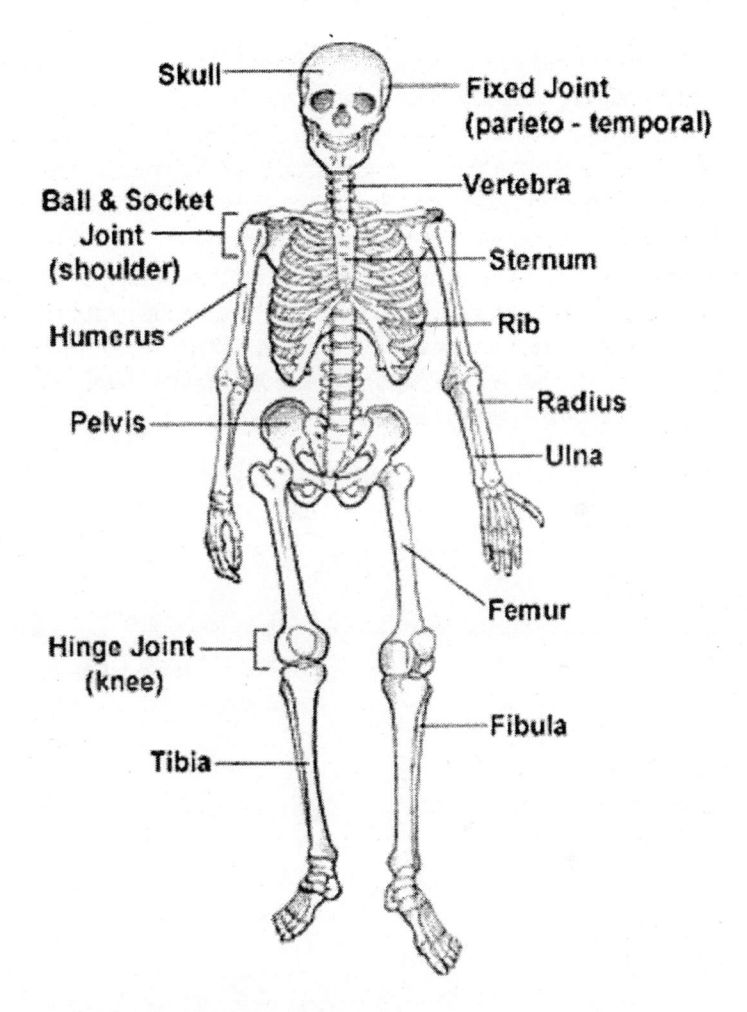

- Skull
- Fixed Joint (parieto - temporal)
- Ball & Socket Joint (shoulder)
- Vertebra
- Sternum
- Humerus
- Rib
- Pelvis
- Radius
- Ulna
- Femur
- Hinge Joint (knee)
- Fibula
- Tibia

an extra pair of ribs, lying above the normal top pair. These cervical ribs may cause problems by compressing nerves or arteries running into the arm. Lying over the upper ribs of the back are the two flat shoulder blades, and these are also supported, from the front, by the two collar bones which link the top of the sternum, on each side, to a bony process on each scapula. Without the scapulas and clavicles we would have no shoulders.

This incomplete ring of bones is called the shoulder girdle. Each scapula bears on its upper and outer angle, a shallow cavity in which the head of the upper arm bone sits. Because the cavity is so shallow, movement of the arm at the shoulder can occur in an arc of 360 degrees. The bottom end of the humerus joins with the forearm bones, the radius and ulna and the bottom ends of these with the eight carpal bones of the wrist. Beyond these are the five metacarpals of the palm of the hand and the fourteen phalanger of the fingers and thumb. Each finger has three phalanges; the thumb has two.

5

Nervous System

In humans, it consists of the central and peripheral nervous systems, the former consisting of the brain and spinal cord and the latter of the nerves, which carry impulses to and from the central nervous system. The cranial nerves handle head and neck sensory and motor activities, except the vagus nerve, which conducts signals to visceral organs. Each spinal nerve is attached to the spinal cord by a sensory and a motor root. These exit between the vertebrae and merge to form a large mixed nerve, which branches to supply a defined area of the body. Disorders include amyotrophic lateral sclerosis, chorea, epilepsy, myasthenia gravis, neural tube defect, parkinsonism, and poliomyelitis. Effects of disorders range from transient tics and minor personality changes to major personality disruptions, seizures, paralysis, and death.

Nervous systems are of two general types, diffuse and centralized. In the diffuse type of system, found in lower invertebrates, there is no brain, and neurons are distributed throughout the organism in a netlike pattern. In the centralized systems of higher invertebrates and vertebrates, a portion of the nervous system has a dominant role in coordinating information and directing responses. This centralization reaches its culmination in vertebrates, which have a well-developed brain and spinal cord. Impulses are carried to and from the brain and spinal cord by nerve fibres that make up the peripheral nervous system.

NEURO-TRANSMITTERS

A neuro-transmitter is a chemical substance selectively released from a nerve ending by the arrival of a nerve impulse. The neuro-transmitter then interacts with a receptor on an adjacent structure to trigger off some kind of response. The adjacent structure may be another nerve, a muscle fibre or a gland. Nerve action, mediated by neuro-transmitters, is a sensitive process that can be increased or decreased as needed. And because the chemical structure of many of the neuro-transmitters is known, they can be used as drugs to modulate some of the most important actions of the nervous system.

In addition, many highly effective drugs act by simulating the action of neuro-transmitters, by modifying their action or by blocking the receptor sites at which they normally act. The main neuro-transmitters are acetylcholine, dopamine, noradrenaline, serotonin, GABA, the endorphins, the enkephalins, glycine, glutamate, aspartine, adrenaline, histamine, vasopressin and bradykinin.

NEURONS

The nervous system consists of an enormous collection of interconnected neurons. Each neuron is a single nerve cell consisting of a cell body, a long nerve fibre or axon, running out of it, and one, or usually more, shorter nerve processes, known as dendrites, running into the nerve body. The cell body contains the nucleus. Neurons interconnect with each other at specialized junctions called synapses and, at most of these, activity is transmitted by release of chemical messengers called neuro-transmitters. Synapses occur mainly between the end of the axon of one neuron and the cell body or the dendrites of another, but may occur between dendrities and axons. Many neurons receive up to 15,000 synapses and some more than 100,000 and the great majority are inter-neurons connecting with other nerve cells, rather than with muscles or glands. This arrangement allows for a system of transmission of nerve impulses, some executory, some inhibitory, which can operate similarly to electronic 'gates' in computers and by which all logical functions may be performed.

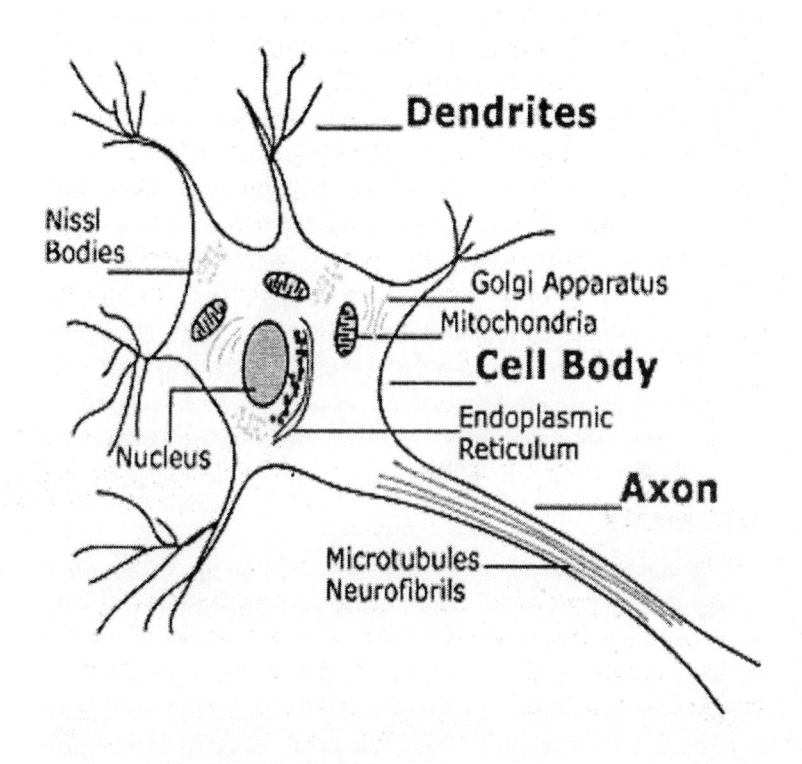

The same arrangement, assuming a constant circulation of nerve impulses, provides a physical basis for any from of memory, whether consciously recallable or of the form equivalent to the software in the read-only memory of a computer. The network of neurons is functionally, and structurally, affected by past experience and experience causes the brain to acquire greater complexity of the branching pattern of dendrites, an increase in the number of supporting cells and changes in the structure and ease of firing of synapses. The ability of the brain to change with experience is called plasticity and although plasticity in some areas, some as those concerned with vision, is lost by about the age of seven, in others it persists throughout life. Brain neuron connections which have not been challenged by experience retain simpler patterns and lower functional capacity.

THE BRAIN

Weighing about three pounds, the brain contains a staggering number of nerve cells and connecting fibres. The packing density, in terms of functional elements, is still several times that of the most compact of electronic computer hardware and no present computer can challenge the capacity of the brain, weight for weight. The neurological organization of all the millions of interconnected nerves of the brain forms of computing system broadly equivalent to many thousands of electronic microcomputers, working in parallel but with extensive interconnections.

The arrangement of parallel computing is the principle difference between the brain and most present-day electronic computers, which are essentially serial and carry out only one operation at a time. It is probable the future research will show that the positive, as well as the negative, characteristics of human intelligence, memory and other functions are essentially those of a parallel computing system. As a result, we may soon need computer psychiatrists. The brain is the information centre of the body, the seat of consciousness and pleasure. It is the physical data store and retains, in a form suitable for mass storage, all the significant individual experience and learning from birth–a unique collection of data which underlies the whole personality and capability of the individual.

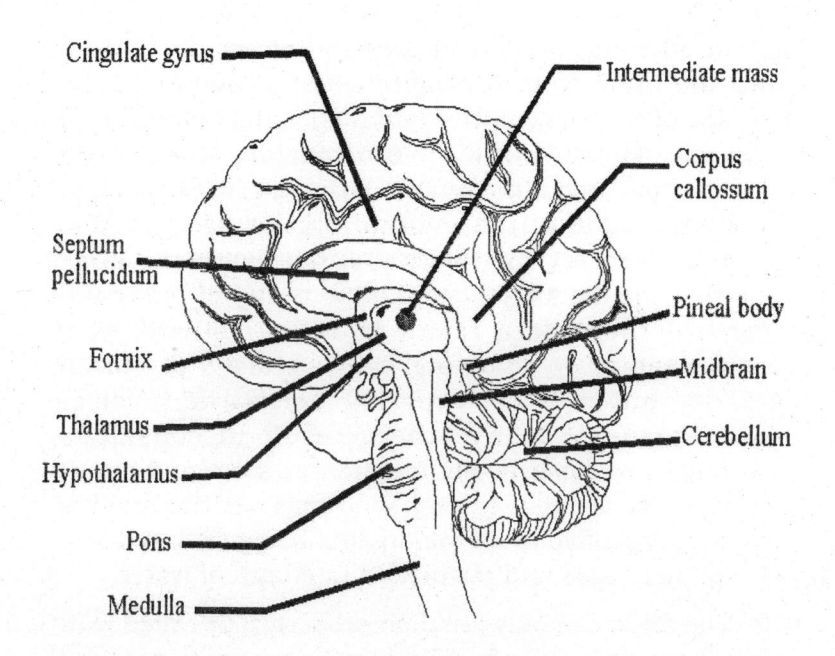

The brain also includes a great deal of data in the form of inherited information such as instincts, patterns of response, and so on. It is probable that the brain cannot function unless continuously supplied with incoming stimuli. The receptors of the four main information modalities are connected directly to the brain by input channels in the form of short nerve tracts–the optic nerves, the auditory nerves, the olfactory nerves and the glossopharyngeal nerves. A constant barrage of data passes in by these nerves and is analysed, coordinated with existing stored data, stored and, if necessary, acted upon.

In addition, a mass of sensory information comes into the brain from specialized nerve endings in the surface of the skin, in the muscles, joints and internal organs. These supply information about the environment, about the relative position of the limbs and about the state of the internal organs. Most of this incoming sensory information is relayed in the large nucleus, the thalamus, deep in the centre of the brain. Many of these data result in reflex activity, of a compensatory or adjusting kind, mediated by brain activity but mostly occurring below the level of consciousness. Many others result in conscious awareness of some bodily function or state and result in voluntary action. For very good reasons, the brain is the best protected of all the organs, being enclosed in a strong bony case and cushioned in a bath of water.

The brain can only function properly if provided with an unceasing supply of sugar, oxygen and other nutrients by way of the bloodstream and to this end it has by far the most profuse blood supply of any organ. Two large arteries, the carotids, run up the front of the neck to the brain and two others, the vertebras, run up through a chain of holes in the side processes of the bones of the neck. These four vessels run into a circle of arteries at the base of the brain, from which major branches arise and run into the substance of the brain itself. The main mass of the brain is called the cerebrum and consists of two, almost mirror-image, cerebral hemispheres largely separated from each other but connected by a massive multi-cable junction called the corpus callosum.

Tucked under the surface of the cerebrum, at the back, lies the cerebellum, or hind-brain, a smaller structure concerned mainly with unconscious and automatic functions such as balance and the control and coordination of voluntary movements. Running down from the middle of the under side of the cerebrum, just in front of the cerebellum, is the brain stem, a thick stalk containing the roots of most of the twelve pairs of nerves which emerge directly from the brain. The brain stem is continuous with the spinal cord, below, and also contains the great tracts of nerve fibres running up and down, into and out of the spinal cord, which connect the brain to the rest of the body, carrying electrical impulses to cause the muscles to contract, and sensory information upwards from all regions to the brain.

THE CELLULAR STRUCTURE OF THE NERVOUS SYSTEM

On microscopic examination, the nerve centres reveal an astonishingly intricate structure consisting of nerve cells and their branches. A neuron is a nerve cell including its branches, and the whole nervous system is made up of neurons. Most nerve cells have two kinds of branches, a single axon and many dendrities. The dendrites are short tree-like branches, while the axon, though very slender, may be inches or feet in length. The axon, as was said before, is the core of a nerve fibre.

The axons in the motor nerves are outgrowths of nerve cells in the cord and brain stem; each motor axon extends from some part of the gray matter of the cord or brain stem out to some muscle. It receives stimuli from the gray matter and conducts nerve currents out to it muscle where it arouses a small squad of muscle fibres to activity. The axons of the optic nerve are branches of nerve cells in the retina, and extend into the brain stem. Light entering the eyes and falling on the retina excites nerve currents which pass back along the axons of the optic nerve to a lower centre in the brain stem and thence to the cerebrum. The olfactory axons are branches of sense cells in the nose.

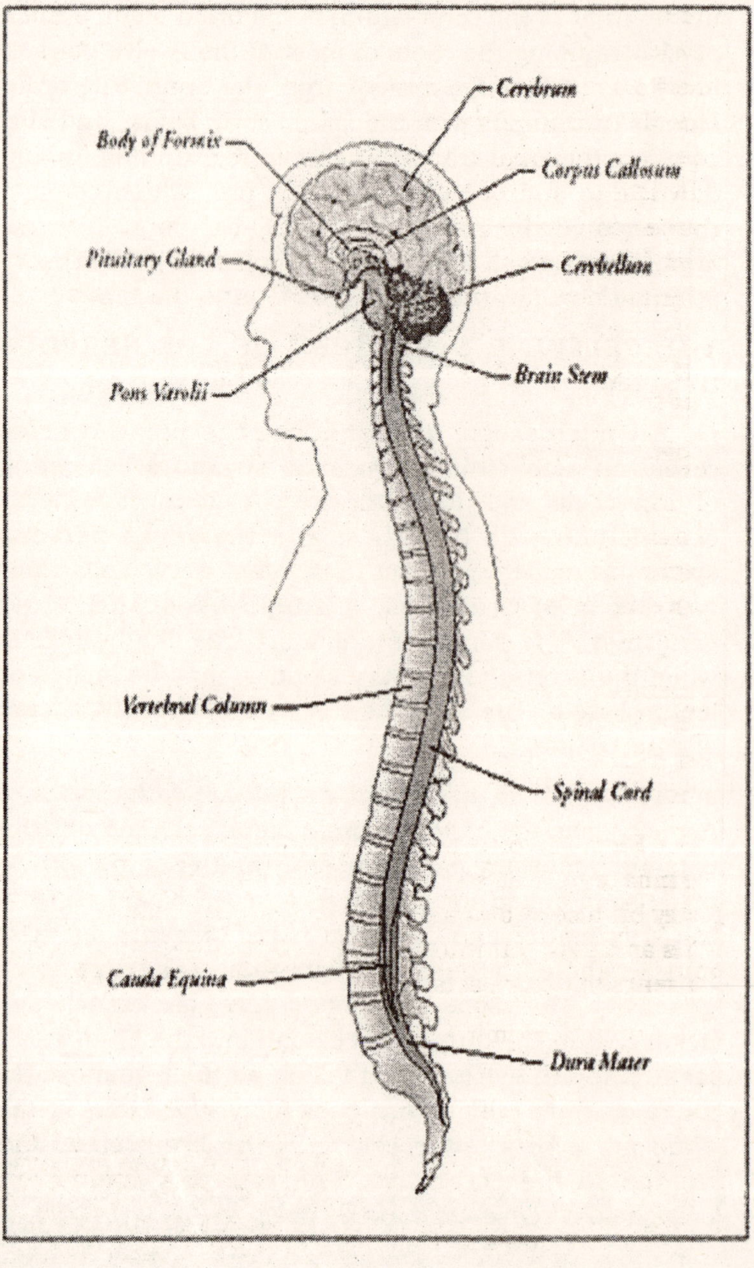
Cerebrum
Body of Fornix
Corpus Callosum
Pituitary Gland
Cerebellum
Pons Varolii
Brain Stem
Vertebral Column
Spinal Cord
Cauda Equina
Dura Mater

The axons of all the other sensory nerves are branches of nerve cells which lie in little bunches close beside the cord and brain stem, and which, by exception, have no dendrites but bifurcated axons extending in one direction outward to the skin or other sense organ and in the other direction inward to the gray matter of the cord or brain stem, thus providing a path from the sense organ to the lower centres. The dendrites are short and do not extend beyond the gray matter where their cells are located. Gray matter consists of nerve cells and their dendrites, and of the tip ends of axons which have grown into a particular bit of the gray matter and broken up there into fine branches.

Inferences from brain structure to brain function

Starting from the assumption that cortical activity consists of nerve currents moving through nerve cells, axons and dendrities, we can hazard some reasonable conjectures based on the facts of brain structure.

- This impression is strengthened when we consider that these numerous interlacing branches are not hard twigs like those of an undergrowth of bushes in a jungle, but delicate soft structures growing or living in a watery medium.

- Each bit of cortex shows incoming axons which terminate in that bit and bring in nerve currents; and every bit also shows axons which emerge from the local cells and pass out into the white matter, carrying nerve currents to other parts of the brain and cord.

- by its incoming projection fibres, a bit of cortex receives stimuli from the lower centres which themselves receive stimuli from the sense organs. By its outgoing projection fibres, the cortex stimulates the lower centres which in turn stimulate the muscles and glands.

- With so much intimate contact between adjacent

neurons it does not seem possible that they can act separately. The whole arrangement seems to insure that they act in "squads, companies and regiments," as said before.

- Besides dividing these axon connections of any bit of cortex into the incoming and the outgoing, we can divide them into "projection" and "association" fibres. The projection fibres lead to or from the lower centres in the brain stem and cord, while the association fibres lead from one part of the cortex to another, a large body of them leading from one hemisphere to the other by way of the "corpus callosum."

- Thus the internal structure of the brain leads to the conclusion (a) that adjacent neurons act together, (b) that non-adjacent parts of the cortex, interconnected by association adjacent parts of the cortex, interconnected by association fibres, also act together, and (c) that the cerebrum, cerebellum and lower centres, all being interconnected by projection fibres, act together. It should be added that the lower centres themselves are interconnected by nerve fibres. When we try to picture how the nervous system performs its part in any activity of the individual, we have to avoid two opposite errors.

First, the activity of the nervous system at any time cannot be confined to single neurons, to single chains of neurons, or even to any one small local centre. The interconnections are so rich that the isolated action of small bits is almost impossible.

Second, it is equally false to say that the cerebrum "acts as a whole." In view of the close connections of cerebrum, cerebellum and lower centres, the statement should at any rate be broadened to read that the nervous system acts as a whole. This more comprehensive statement, however, fails to take into account the elaborate structure of the nervous system, with its definite fibre paths leading from one particular part to another particular part.

The connection of the cortex with the lower centres, by way of the projection fibres, differ from one part of the cortex to another; and though the association fibres are not easily disentangled, it is certain that neighbouring parts are in general more richly connected than distant parts, that corresponding parts of the two hemispheres are closely tied together, and that in short the association fibres provide specific rather than merely diffuse connections. Another objection to saying that the nervous system acts as a whole is that if we mean "as a whole" literally, we are saying that every single neuron in the whole system is acting at once. Then, according to the all or none law, every neuron is acting full strength. Therefore every action of the nervous system would be the same as every other; the organism could do only one thing and that would amount to a general convulsion. It is certain that the brain performs many different acts, and that no two of them can be performed with exactly the same combination of neurons. The theory to which we are led is treat the brain acts in patterns, and that the patterns must often involve many different parts of the cortex as well as parts of the lower centres.

The Synapse

It is in the gray matter that neurons are interconnected. Formerly they were supposed to grow together into a network of cytoplasm, through which nerve currents could pass freely in any direction. But this old "nerve net" conception gave way to the "neuron theory," now thoroughly established. The neurons begin their careers in prenatal life as little separate round cells, without branches, and latter send out axon and dendrites; and though they establish close contacts with each other by these branches, they never fuse, but each neuron always remains a separate cell. This form of connection, by contact and not by growing together, is called synaptic connection, and the contact between one neuron and another is called a synapse. For simplicity let us first consider just two neurons and their synaptic connection.

The axon of one neuron breaks up into an end-brush of fine branches, which interlace with the dendrites of the other neuron. In some cases, however, the end-brush of the first neuron envelops the cell body of the second neuron. In the either case the contact is close enough to enable the first neuron to stimulate the second. The dendrite in a synapse is a receiving organ, while the axon end-brush is a stimulator and not a receiver. What happens at the synapse, then, is that the end-brush of one neuron stimulates the dendrities of another neuron. Communication across a synapse is always in one direction, from the end-brush of one neuron to the dendrites of another. Though the contact between neurons at the synapse is close, it is not always and everywhere equally close. Some synapses are visible closer than others, and it is probable that the resistance of the same synapse varies from time to time, with the condition of the blood, with activity and fatigue and perhaps with repeated exercise or training. It can readily be seen that the synapse is an attractive idea to play with in theorizing as to the physiology of behaviour, but one has to admit that the actual happenings in this minute arrangement are only vaguely understood at present. One misconception that might be created by our simplified diagram should be corrected at once. Single synapses, if they occur, are the exception; multiple synapses are the rule.

In any small region of gray matter, several axons can be found terminating in end-brushes, and the cells of that region receive stimulation from all these axons, which may have come from quite different parts. The large motor neurons of the cord, which directly control the muscles, are acted on by axons from the local sensory nerves, by axons from various parts of the cord and brain stem, and by axons from the cerebrum—all of which have a share in determining whether or not the motor neuron shall be activated and whether or not the connected muscle fibres shall contract. Any give nerve cell is likely to be acted on by several other neurons, and also to act upon several others.

THE NERVE CENTRE

We sometimes speak of many nerve centres, but they are all interconnected and are included within the one big centre consisting of the brain and spinal cord. The brain lies in the skull and the cord extends from the base of the brain down through a tube in the vertebral column or backbone. We may think of the brain as consisting of three main parts: the brain stem and the two great outgrowths from the brain stem known as the cerebrum and the cerebellum. The brain stem and spinal cord, taken together, are the axis of the whole nervous system. This axis is connected with the sense organs by the sensory nerves and with the muscles and glands by the motor nerves, while it is also connected by great bundles of nerve fibres with the cerebrum and cerebellum. The nerves of the arms, legs and most of the trunk connect with the cord, while the head and face nerves connect with the brain stem, as do also the nerves of the lungs, heart and stomach.

We may speak of the cord as containing the "lower centres" for the limbs and of the brain stem as containing the lower centres for the face, mouth, lungs, etc. The "higher centre" in the cerebrum and cerebellum act upon these lower centres and are acted on by them, and it is only through the intermediary of the lower centres that the higher or with the environment. The lower centres are masses of gray matter lying inside the cord and brain stem, while the higher centres consist of gray matter lying on the surface of the cerebrum and cerebellum and forming the cortex of these structures.

The remaining fifty percent of the brain and cord is white matter, which consists of nerve fibres linking together all parts of the gray matter, just as the nerves consist of fibres linking the lower centres with the muscles and sense organs. Like the body, the nervous system is divisible into bilaterally symmetrical halves, and in the cerebrum the right and left halves are called the cerebral hemispheres. It is a curious fact that the nerve fibres connecting the hemispheres with the lower centres cross or "decussate" so that the left hemisphere is connected with the right side of the brain stem and cord and through them with the right side of the body. The right hand and the left hemisphere work together.

THE NERVES

But the organism would be a sluggish hulking sort of unit without the third integrating system consisting of rapidly conducting nerves. A general view of the nervous system shows nerves ramifying to every nook and corner of the body. But a second glance shows that no part is directly connected with any other, for the nerves radiate from the brain and spinal cord. These two central masses are continuous with each other and constitute the nerve centre, and all the nerves lead to or from this big general centre. The sensory nerves conduct into the centre and the motor nerves out from the centre.

A touch on the skin starts nerve currents which run

Nervous System

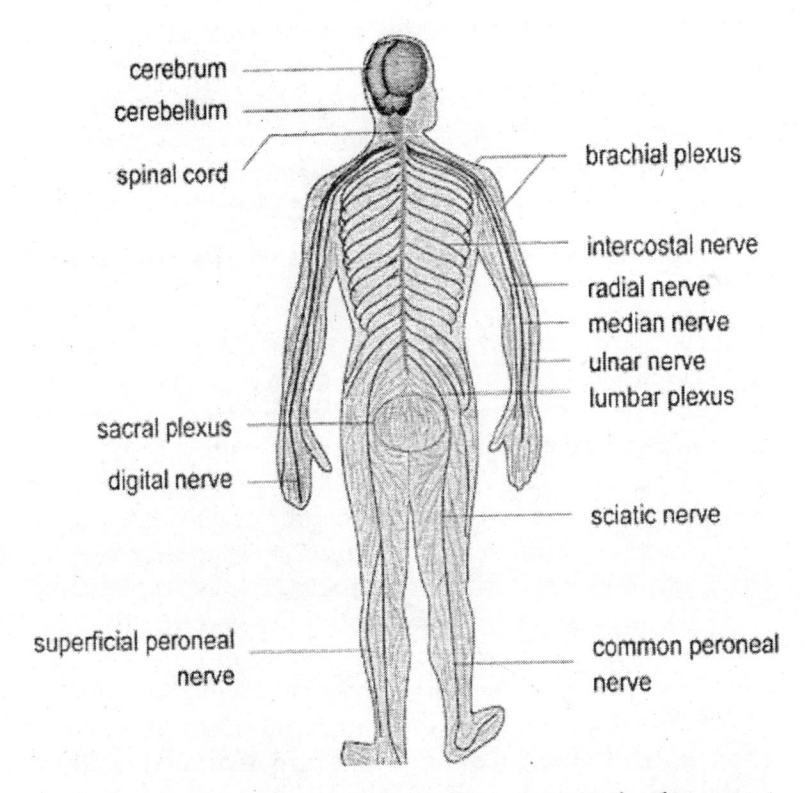

Diagram labels: cerebrum, cerebellum, spinal cord, sacral plexus, digital nerve, superficial peroneal nerve, brachial plexus, intercostal nerve, radial nerve, median nerve, ulnar nerve, lumbar plexus, sciatic nerve, common peroneal nerve

along a sensory nerve to the centre. Activity in the nerve centre starts currents out along the motor nerves to the muscles. The advantage of having all the organs tied to a common centre is obvious: the organism is able to act as a unity.

The nerve current

What is it that the nerves conduct? We call it the nerve current, and as far as known it is an electro-chemical wave motion, very weak and consuming very little energy, but capable of arousing a muscle or a nerve centre to action. The nerve current travels along the nerve at the fairly respectable speed of something like 100 yards a second. The waves in different motor nerves are the same in nature and produce different motor effects simply because the nerves lead to different muscles. All nerve currents are fundamentally alike. The nerve fibre is a conductor, and that is all. Stimulated at one end, it passes the stimulation along to the structure with which it is connected at the other end.

The nervous system compared with a telephone system

If the circulation is a transportation system, carrying materials, the nervous system, carrying messages or stimuli, has some analogy with the telephone system of a town. Both take up little space and consume little fuel. The nerves are like telephone cables in being bundles of insulated conductors, each conductor leading to a separate point outside but all converging to a common centre where connections are made. The nerve centre, like some telephone centrals, is essentially an automatic switchboard, but the operation of the nerve centre is very different from that of any other switchboard. The connections made are multiple rather than single. One incoming calls are switched to the same outgoing line, and all the calls at any one time are interconnected. The nerve centre is an integrating switch board.

Nerve fibres

Even a slender nerve contains many nerve fibres, and the largest nerve in the body, the optic nerve conducting from the eye to the brain, contains up to 400,000 of them. Each nerve fibres is a fine thread, microscopic in thickness but long enough to reach from its sense organ or muscle to the nerve centre. The single nerve fibre, like an insulated wire, has a core surrounded by a sheath. The core, called the axon, is a branch of a nerve cell, as well shall soon see. Though so

Nervous System

very fine, the axon breaks up into still finer branches where it terminates in a sense organ or muscle, and it is these delicate nerve ends that receive the stimulus in the case of a sensory fibre, and that stimulate a muscle or gland in the case of a motor fibre.

THE VISUAL AREA

Man's eyes, placed side by side and looking forward, get almost the same view; both have nearly the same "field of vision." On account of the crossing of the rays of light within the eyeball, light from an object in the right half of the field of view, at the right of the momentary fixation point, falls on the left half of the retina, light from the upper part of the field of view falls on the lower part of the retina; and this is true for both eyes alike. The central part of each retina is specially well developed and provides the most distinct vision; it receives the light from the object "looked at," i.e., from the fixation point and the central part of the field of view. Since we "see single, not double," most of the time, it is clear that the brain must somehow integrate the messages received from the two eyes. Probably, one would guess, the nerve fibres leading to the brain from corresponding parts of the two retains get together somewhere.

Varieties of blindness

The results of fibre tracing can be checked by studying the losses of vision resulting from known injuries to different parts of the nerve apparatus. If the optic nerve is severed between one eye and the chiasm, that eye is of course completely blind, the other not affected. If the nerve is cut behind the chiasm, on the right side, the left half of the field of view is lost for both eyes alike.

This hemianopsia is what we should expect from the results of fibre tracing. The same left-sided hemianopsia

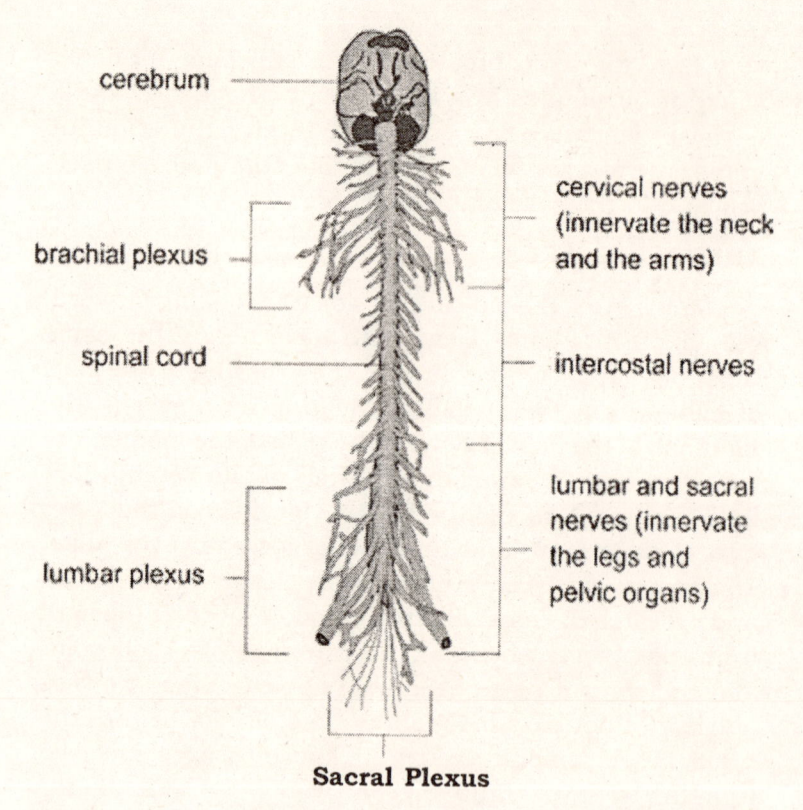

![Diagram of the central nervous system with labels: cerebrum, brachial plexus, spinal cord, lumbar plexus, cervical nerves (innervate the neck and the arms), intercostal nerves, lumbar and sacral nerves (innervate the legs and pelvic organs), Sacral Plexus]

occurs when the injury has destroyed the right lower visual centre, or the pathway thence to the right area striata, or the right striata itself. The right hemisphere does see the left half of the field of view, etc., as was predicted from the fibre connections. In this way vision is brought into line with body sensation and movement, in which the right hemisphere has to do with the left side of the body.

Effect of stimulating the visual area

Though the results and conclusions stated have obtained the general acceptance of experts, it must not be thought that it was a simple matter to obtain the cleancut case material necessary. Numerous cases of gunshot and shrapnel wounds during the World War helped greatly towards what seems now to be a final decision on the main points. There is still another line of evidence which is striking and convincing. When the skull has to be opened up and the occipital lobe exposed to view for the removal of a tumour, a weak electric current can be applied to points on the cortex and the subject asked to report his experience we might hastily assume that he would report pain, on the supposition that the brain must be very "sensitive." But no, stimulation of the visual area ought to give some visual sensation.

One leading student of these matters reports the following results in one especially clear case: stimulation at the occipital pole caused the subject to see a bright light straight in front; applied to the upper part of the visual area it caused him to see a flickering something down below, and applied to the lower part of the area it gave the same only in the upper part of the field of view. These localizations correspond to the results obtained by the other methods. When the electric stimulus was applied outside the area striata but on neighbouring parts of the occipital lobe, the subject reported more complex visual appearances: flames, stars, shiny balls, butterflies, various objects and even persons.

It would seem then that a large share of the occipital lobe had to do with vision. The area striata, which receives the nerve currents from the retina, undoubtedly passes the stimulation along by association fibres to the neighbouring regions, and the latter contribute to the perception and understanding of what is seen. Injuries to the occipital region, if not involving the area striata, are found to produce, not blindness, but inability to recognize objects, or to read, or to distinguish colours, or to find one's way be the sense of sight.

Other Sensory Areas of the Cortex

Similar work has been done on the other senses and similar results obtained. Each sense has a lower centre in or adjacent to that part of the brain stem known as the thalamus. Incoming fibres which pass to the several sensory areas of the cortex. Destruction of the auditory area in both hemispheres makes the individual deaf, and destruction of any part of the somesthetic areas abolishes sensation in some part of the body.

Fibre Tracing

The optic nerves, passing back from the eyes, come together and separate again, forming an X which is called the optic chiasm, after the Greek letter Chi. Behind the chiasm they diverge right and left and terminate in the lower visual centres in the brain stem. Masses of nerve fibres emerge from the lower visual centre of the right side, pass into the right hemisphere and turn back into the occipital lobe. So much is relatively easy anatomy; but to trace these nerve fibres to their termination very painstaking methods are needed. One such is the degeneration methods.

When a nerve fibre is separated from its own nerve cell it degenerates and so can be traced. If the right eye is destroyed, the entire right optic nerve degenerates back to the chiasm, but from there back to the brain stem the degenerated fibre are divided about equally between the two nerves and so between the two lower visual centres. If the eye injury affects only the right side of the retina the degenerated fibres all go back to the lower visual centre of the right side. Thus the nerve fibres from the right halves of both eyes come together in the lower visual centre of the right side; and similarly, left to left. With an injury to the retina, the degenerated fibres end in the lower visual centres; but if one of these lower centres is itself destroyed, degenerated fibres can be traced thence into the occipital lobe, where they all terminate in a limited region of cortex known as the area striata or striped area, because of the peculiar stratification of its cells.

The area striata is, indeed, one of the best marked of the regions in the anatomical map of the cortex. It lies mostly on the mesial surface of the hemisphere, facing the other hemisphere, and extends from the occipital pole of the cerebrum forward for a couple of inches on this mesial surface. The fibre-tracing method, accordingly, locates the cortical visual area in the area striata. It locates the visual area for the right half of both retinas in the area striata of the right hemisphere, and for the left in the left. The right hemisphere ought to see what the right half of each retina sees, namely, the left half of the field of view.

Psychological experiments on the occipital lobe

Experiments on trained rats have shown that the habit of entering a door marked by a white square or any other particular shape is lost when the occipital lobes are removed and that it cannot be re-learned, whereas loss of other parts of the cortex does not interfere with this visual recognition of shape. Distinguishing between lights of differing brightness also depends on the occipital lobe, though not quite to the same extent as discrimination of shapes. Light can be distinguished from darkness by the rat, however, even after the occipital lobes have been removed, though if the animal has learned in the intact condition to enter a lighted door and avoid a dark one, he loses the habit when the occipital lobes are removed.

It would seem from these results that the rat can get along with only his lower visual centres when it is only a question of distinguishing light from dark, but that more precise use of visual data requires the presence of some amount of occipital cortex. Man is more dependent on his cortex than the rat, and is absolutely blind if the occipital lobe is lost from both hemispheres. One characteristic of the higher mammals, and especially of man, is the great size of the cerebrum in comparison with the brains stem. Functions that are performed by the brain stem in lower forms have been shift to the cerebrum in man.

THE ASSOCIATION AREAS OR INTEGRATING AREAS

With the sensory and motor areas identified, there still remains a large fraction not the cortex unaccounted for, especially in the human brain. There is one large area lying in the parietal, temporal and occipital lobes, intervening between the several sensory areas; and there is another in the frontal lobe forward of the motor and pre-motor areas. These are called association areas, on the theory that they serve to combine or integrate the activities of the sensory and motor areas. Their function is thus supposed to be synthetic. The evidence regarding them comes mostly from cases of brain injury in man. The functional losses resulting from such injuries are classed under several heads.

Apraxia

Apraxia, or loss of ability to "do," is akin to aphasia. A test consists in giving the individual a box of matches and a cigar; he may be unable to make the right combinations, though perfectly capable of making all the necessary single movements. The injury varies in location, but is usually not far from the motor area, either in from or behind.

Agnosia

Agnosia, or loss of ability to "know" or perceive.

Visual agnosia was alluded to before in connection with the occipital lobes; it consists in inability to recognize objects, words, shapes and colours. In auditory agnosia, sounds cannot be recognized, or music cannot be followed and appreciated as before. The injury here is in the neighbourhood of the auditory area. When the injury is close behind the somesthetic area, the subject cannot recognize objects placed in his hands, judge weights by lifting them, etc. In an agnosia the subject still sees, hears or feels, but he cannot utilize the sensory data as signs of definite objective facts.

Aphasia

Aphasia is a loss or disturbance of speech, and occurs in several different forms. Through brain injury and individual may become unable to hear speech with any understanding, or unable to in the right words to express his meaning, though he may speak fluently; as one old gentleman mystified his friends by asserting that he "must go and have his umbrella washed," till it was discovered that he wanted his hair cut. The brain injury in such cases as the above is likely to be in the neighbourhood of the auditory area. In other cases the great difficulty is to get the words out, some subjects being able to speak only one or two words of very frequent usage, while others can pronounce separate words but cannot put them together into sentences. In this class of cases the injury is apt to be in the pre-motor area, a part of which has long been known as the motor speech centre, though of late years it has been regarded with some scepticism.

LOCALIZED AND UNLOCALIZED BRAIN FUNCTIONS

Since different parts of the nervous system differ in structure and have different connections, it is a fair guess that they play different roles in the activity of the organism. This question has been much to the fore ever since about 1800, when Gall propounded his theory of phrenology, a theory which had a vast popular vogue though it never received any scientific support. Gall himself, however, was a scientific anatomist of standing. His method of study was a primitive sort of correlation. When he noticed an individual with a peculiar shape of head, he tried to ascertain his mental peculiarities, so as to tie up different mental and behaviour characteristics with different elevations and depressions in the external surface of the skull, from which he believed it possible to infer the degree of development of the underlying brain parts. The intellectual faculties he placed in the front part of the brain, within the forehead, moral characteristics in about the middle, and the animal propensities in the rear, sex desire for example in the cerebellum.

MATURATION AND EXERCISE IN THE DEVELOPMENT OF THE NERVOUS SYSTEM

There is abundant evidence of maturation. The first rudiment of the nervous system appears when the embryo is about two weeks old. A longitudinal groove appears in the outer layer of cells in the region that is to become the back, and this groove shortly closes over and forms a tube. These developments so far are a response of one part of the embryo to the influence of adjoining parts, and not to external stimulation. The metabolic activity is greatest at the head end of the embryo, and that end of the neural tube develops most rapidly and most elaborately, so that at the early age of four weeks of embryonic life the main parts of the brain are distinguishable. In these early stages, the cells composing the rudimentary brain and cord are not neurons, but as the cells multiply, they come to have the character of nerve cells, and send out first their axons and later their dendrites.

The motor neurons and nerves develop earlier than the sensory. The brain develops early, and the cerebral cortex shows growing nerve cells, with axons and dendrites, long before this portion of the nervous system can be participating in the simple activities of the fetus. It is clear from these facts that the general form, structure and characteristics of the brain develop by maturation.

Evidence for growth of the nervous system through its activity is less clear, but there is evidence. Though no new neurons are formed after birth, growth of the nerve cell and of its branches continues rapidly in early childhood and more slowly on into adult life. This growth need not be entirely due to activity but activity is probably one stimulating factor. In the area striata, which certainly is active enough after birth, the nerve cells increase in size up to the age of eight years and apparently to some extent even later.

THE REFLEX ARC

In the intact organism the lower and higher centres work intimately together; but the lower can operate to a certain extent even when separated from the higher. Transection of the spinal cord, separating the lower part completely from the brain, occurs by accident or in an animal experiment. A pinch applied to one hind paw still gives a quick response called the "flexion reflex" by which that paw is pulled up while the opposite leg is thrust downward. This reflex ceases if the lower part of the cord is destroyed or its nerves cut. A reflex is a prompt muscular or glandular response to a sensory stimulus, an involuntary and unlearned response.

A local reflex is one obtainable from a fraction of the whole organism. The machinery that carries out a reflex includes a sensory nerve entering the gray matter of the cord or brain stem, and a motor nerve issuing from this gray matter and leading to the responding muscles. A minimum diagram of this reflex mechanism shows a sensory axon leading into the gray matter of a lower centre and forming synaptic connection there with a motor neuron whose axon extends out to the muscle.

A Reflex Arc Shows How Neuron Types Work Together.

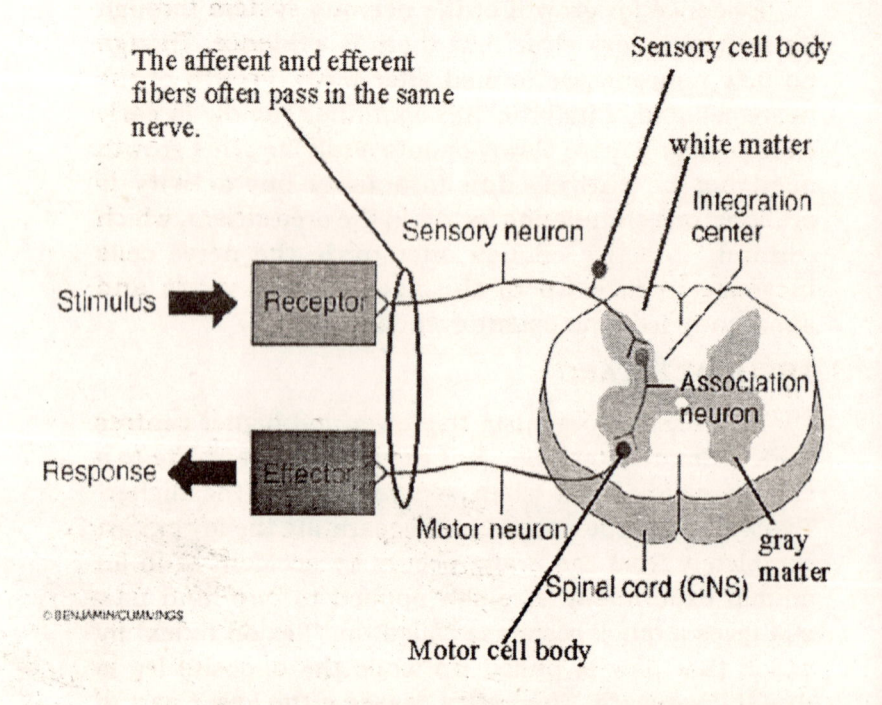

Diagram labels: The afferent and efferent fibers often pass in the same nerve. Sensory cell body. Sensory neuron. white matter. Integration center. Stimulus → Receptor. Association neuron. Response ← Effector. Motor neuron. Spinal cord (CNS). gray matter. Motor cell body.

This combination of a sensory and a motor neuron makes up a two-neuron "reflex arc." A three-neuron arc is the minimum diagram for breathing, which can go on in the absence of the brain, provided the lower part of the brain stem and the upper part of the cord, with their nerves, remain intact. Such local reflexes were once regarded as the fundamentals of motor activity, and the organism's behaviour was supposed to consist in combinations of reflexes. The reflex arc was accordingly regarded as picturing the elementary fact in nerve machinery. But there are several objections to this theory.

Converging Paths

The gray matter in any lower or higher centre receives incoming axons from several or many different parts of the nervous system, and is thus subjected to a combination of influences rather than to a single stimulus. The respiratory centre in the brain stem, for example, receives not only sensory nerve currents from the lungs but currents from many or all other sensory nerves as well, so that breathing is instantly modified by a painful stimulus, by a sudden loud noise, or by a dash of cold water on the skin. The respiratory centre also receives nerve fibres from the cerebrum, as we can judge from the fact that the breath can be hastened or slowed voluntarily, and from the modification of breathing that occurs in speaking. Further, the rate and depth of breathing are affected by the amount of carbon dioxide in the blood circulating Through the respiratory centre. So simple three-neuron arc is very far from an adequate picture of the mechanism of breathing.

Facilitation and Inhibition

When two axons from different regions come together into a bit of the gray matter, they facilitate or assist each other's stimulating effect, or they neutralize or inhibit each other's effect. Exactly how inhibition works in the gray matter is not yet known, but one instance of it is afforded by the momentary cessation of breathing when cold is suddenly applied to the skin.

Larger movements not compounds of the local reflexes

Since reflexes are present in the young child, they have been represented as the primary elements from which all motor activity arises by combining them into numerous complex acts. One objection to this conception comes from studying the behaviour of embryos and is to the effect that general movements may antedate local reflexes. The general body movements, then, are not combinations of small local reflexes. The smaller movements appear to differentiate out of the larger.

Branching paths

An adequate picture must show not only converging axons, but also branching axons by which any single neuron can exert its influence upon several other neurons. Thus the nerve currents coming from a single part can be distributed to many parts. The numerous muscle fibres in a single muscle are thus made to act together, and several muscles can be aroused at the same time in a coordinated movement.

Multiple nerve path

Single sensory neurons, and especially single motor neurons, do not act separately. Neurons act in squads, etc., as has been said.

Continued activity

The reflex arc diagram may suggest a nerve centre resting quietly until a particular stimulus arrives—whereas the typical condition of the nerve centre is one of activity. The activity already going on in a nerve centre is modified, facilitated or inhibited, by the incoming nerve currents. We have to think of the nervous system as constantly active, at least during waking hours, as constantly subjected to many varied stimuli and as constantly shifting in its pattern of activity.

THE AUTONOMIC NERVOUS SYSTEM

This is the part of the nervous system which controls functions, such as the heartbeat, the secretion of glands and the contraction of blood vessels, that are not normally under conscious volition. Many automatic and unconscious processes are essential for health and even life, and these are controlled by the autonomic nervous system. It is subdivided into two parts, the sympathetic and the parasympathetic, and these are, in general, contrary and in balance. The sympathetic system arises from the spinal cord in the back and lumbar region and is concerned with the automatic responses of the body to sudden stressful situations.

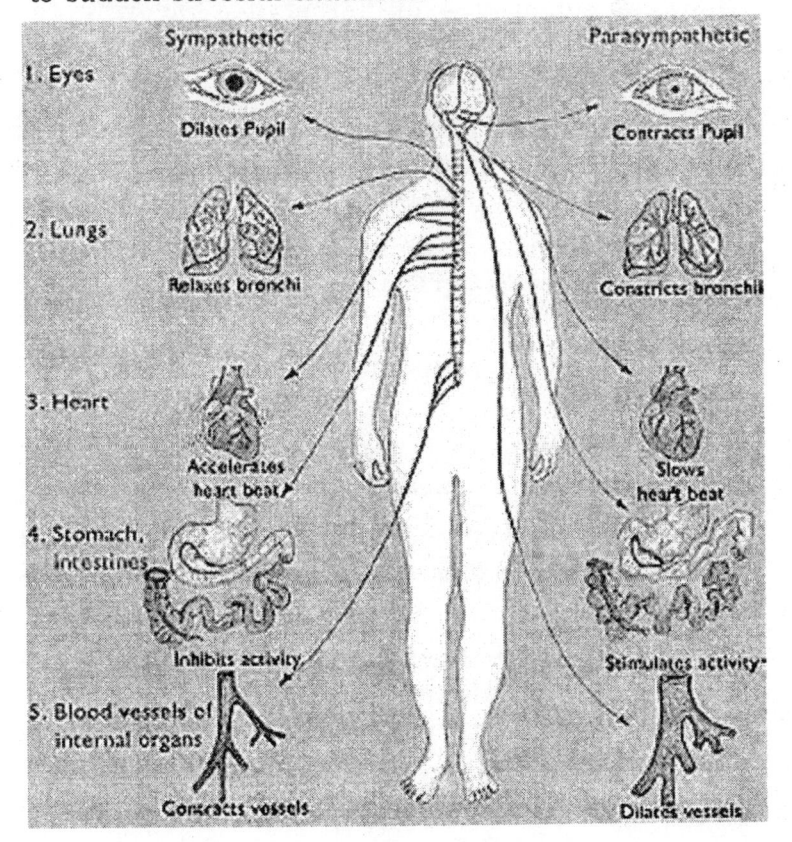

	Sympathetic	Parasympathetic
1. Eyes	Dilates Pupil	Contracts Pupil
2. Lungs	Relaxes bronchi	Constricts bronchii
3. Heart	Accelerates heart beat	Slows heart beat
4. Stomach, intestines	Inhibits activity	Stimulates activity
5. Blood vessels of internal organs	Contracts vessels	Dilates vessels

The autonomic nervous system divides into two parts: the sympathetic nervous system and the parasympathetic nervous system. Both systems are involved with your metabolism and often work in opposition. For example, the sympathetic system is concerned with metabolic processes that use energy. The parasympathetic system is concerned primarily with metabolic processes that conserve energy. In the airways, stimulation of the parasympathetic system causes bronchial tubes to constrict, whereas stimulating the sympathetic nervous system produces the opposite reaction (dilation). In normal airways, a balance between these two systems maintains comfortable breathing. In asthmatic airways, there is sometimes an imbalance favoring the parasympathetic system that produces narrowing or constriction of the airways.

The autonomic nervous system transmits three different types of signals, each of which is handled by a specialized type of receptor.

Alpha receptors recognise the nerve impulses that increase the heart rate, constrict bronchial muscle, and increase mucus production.

Beta-1 receptors increase heart rate and blood pressure.

Beta-2 receptors relax bronchial muscles and decrease mucus production.

Bronchodilators (relievers) are medications that stimulate the Beta-2 receptors, and cause the airways to open.

Recent research has shown that the beta receptors of asthmatics are defective. The parasympathetic nerves of an asthmatic overstimulate the bronchial tubes and this makes the tubes constrict. An overactive parasympathetic nervous system could explain why such nonspecific stimuli such as smoke, viruses and even sudden weather changes trigger wheezing in both allergic and nonallergic asthmatics.

The Cortex

The outer surface of the brain consists mainly of tightly packed nerve cell bodies interconnected by short fibres. The cortex has been accurately mapped out into areas serving known functions such as voluntary movement; sensations of touch; hearing and vision; processing and interpretation of incoming information; and many others. Destruction of these areas, by disease or injury, deprives the individual of the function concerned. The cortex is the seat of the all the higher functions of man–intellectual ability, learning, imagination, social responsibility, altruism, artistic skills, non-sexual love. The 'association areas' of the cortex are areas which although separate from those areas primarily concerned with these various functions, are connected to them by large numbers of nerve fibres.

The association areas are concerned with the integration of input and output data with other aspects of brain function, including memory, and the elaboration of them into the complex processes underlying higher mental functions such as language, imagination and creativity. Thus, damage to the visual association area, while not in any way affecting the primary function of vision, might lead to an inability to recognize or interpret what is seen or might even produce visual hallucinations.

The Meninges and Cerebro-Spinal Fluid

The brain is not entirely formed from nerve and supporting tissue, but contains interconnecting, fluid-filled spaces called ventricles. These also communicate with the cerebro-spinal fluid in which the whole brain and spinal cord are bathed and which fills a narrow duct, the central canal, in the spinal cord. The brain and cord are wrapped in three layers of membrane called the meninges. The inner meninx is a delicate layer, closely applied to the brain and dipping into the grooves on the surface.

This is called the pia mater and the cerebrospinal fluid lies outside it but beneath the next outermost layer, the arachnoid mater. Thus the arachnoid bridges across the grooves in the brain, and the cerebro-spinal fluid is in the space under it. Outermost of all is the tough, fibrous dura mater and this is closely attached to the inside of the skull and the bony canal in the spine in which the spinal cord lies.

The Cranial Nerves

These are the twelve pairs of major nerves arising directly from the brain and brain stem, as distinct from the spinal nerves which emerge from the spinal cord. The cranial nerves are concerned with smell, vision, eye movement, sensation in the head, secretion of tears and saliva, movement of the muscles of facial expression, hearing, tongue movement, chewing and taste. One pair, the vagus nerves, wanders out of the head and travels down as far as the bowels, supplying the heart with rate-control fibres, on the way. All but the first two pairs of the cranial nerves arise from the upper part of the broad stalk of the brain.

The Brain Stem

This is the part of the brain connecting the main masses of the cerebrum and cerebellum, above, with the spinal cord, below. It consists, from above downwards, of the pons and the medulla oblongata and conveys all the large tracts of nerve fibres connecting the brain with the body. The brain stem also contains the roots of the cranial nerves which move the eyes, face and tongue and provide facial sensation, taste and hearing. Most important of all, it contains the net-like radicular formation which is responsible for vital functions such as breathing and heart rate, and which controls and coordinates movement. Brain-stem damage is always very serious and often fatal.

The Hypothalamus

The region of the brain lying near the centre of the under-surface and immediately above the pituitary gland is called the hypothalamus. It consists of three groups of collected nerve cells, including the breastlike pair of mamillary bodies, most of which are connected directly, by nerve fibres, to the pituitary gland, but some of which are connected to other parts of the brain. The hypothalamus is especially important as it is the main point at which the neural hormonal systems of the body interact. Here, electrical brain action, including that governing thought and emotion, causes changes which force the central controlling endocrine gland–the pituitary–to send out chemical messengers to any or all

Diencephalon

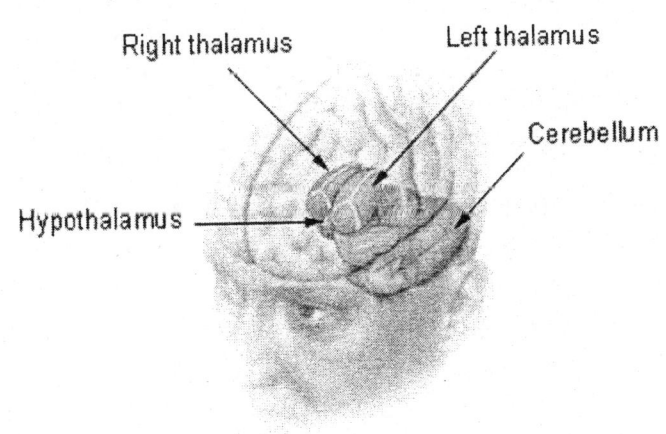

of the other endocrine organs and prompt them into activity.

The result may be the pouring into the bloodstream of hormones such as adrenaline, cortisols, thyroid hormone, sex hormones, milk-secreting hormones and others. All these hormones are associated with changes in the state of the emotions. Baby suckling, for instance, causes the hypothalamus to prompt the pituitary to release the hormone prolactin, which causes the breasts to secrete milk.

The hypothalamus, itself, releases hormones into the blood but these are carried directly to, and act mainly on, the pituitary bland. The hypothalamus constantly receives information from many parts of the body including the blood levels of the various hormones, the current state of bodily and mental stress, the requirements for physical activity and the state of the emotions.

The Cerebellum

This is the smaller subsidiary brain, lying under the rear part of the main brain, the cerebrum, and immediately behind the stalk of the brain. The cerebellum operates at a totally unconscious level and is concerned with the complex task of coordinating the nerve impulses underlying all muscular activity so that smooth, balanced, purposive and effective movements can be made and the body's balance maintained in walking and in other activities. To do this, the cerebellum requires a great deal of information. It must have continuous input:

1. From the eyes, informing it about the environment and the relationship of the body to it;

2. From all the muscles, so that their degree of

contraction is known;

3. From those parts of the main brain concerned with movement.

4. From the balancing mechanisms in the inner ears, conveying information about the position of the head, relative to the different planes, and about accelerative forces experienced by the body;

This nerve-ceasing input of data is passed to the cerebellum by way of large nerve tracts which join it to the brain stem and to several parts of the cerebrum. In the cerebellum the information is automatically coordinated and the complex output to all the muscles, necessary to maintain balanced posture and smooth movement, computed. This output is then passed back to the cerebrum and to the muscles. The study of these effects has taught us much about the function of the cerebellum.

The Peripheral Nerves

Nerves are bundles of neurons, outside the central nervous system, bound together and enclosed in fibrous sheaths. The individual neurons are usually insulated by a layer of white material called myelin, which gives the nerve a white, shiny appearance. Most nerves contain neurons running outward from the central nervous system to all parts of the body and others running from the body inwards to the central nervous system.

The outgoing neurons mostly go to muscles to stimulate them to contract. These neuron bundles are called the motor part of the nerve. Most of the ingoing neuron bundles are carrying information to the brain and from the sensory part of the nerve. So most major nerves are mixed motor and sensory nerves, but near their endings the motor and sensory part separate.

Central Nervous System

Brain

Spinal Cord

Peripheral Nervous System

Peripheral Nerve

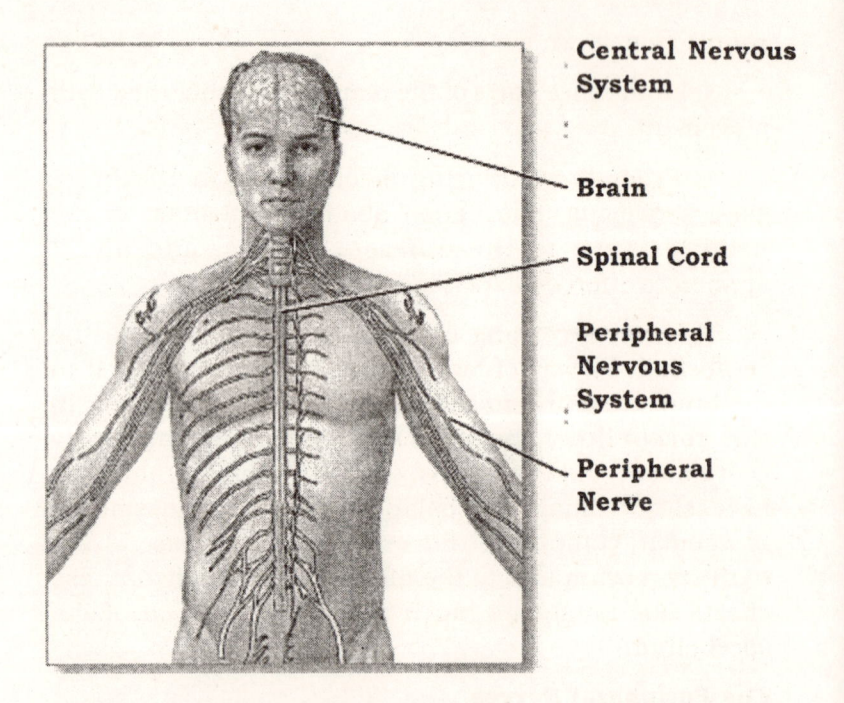

Within the central nervous system neuron bundles from neural tracts. The white matter of the spinal cord and brain consists of many neural tracts. Coming directly from the brain are twelve pairs of cranial nerves, and coming directly from the spinal cord are thirty-one pairs of spinal nerves.

These eighty-six nerves connect to all the muscles in the body and receive information from the whole area of the skin and from all internal organs. A ganglion is a large collection of nerve cell bodies, from which emerges bundles of nerve fibres. Ganglia are present in many parts of the body, some of the most conspicuous being located near the spinal cord and containing the cell bodies of the large spinal nerves entering the cord. Another chain of ganglia, the sympathetic ganglia, lie on either side of the vertebral column, and are linked together by nerve fibres.

Nervous System

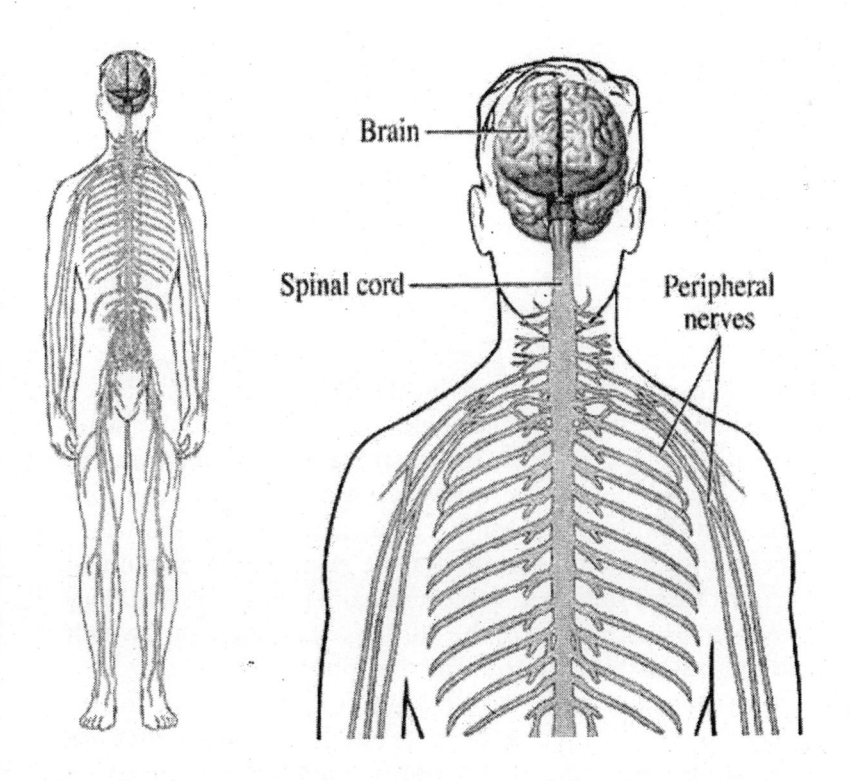

Brain

Spinal cord

Peripheral nerves

6

Circulatory System

The circulatory system is an organ system that passes nutrients (such as amino acids and electrolytes), gases, hormones, blood cells, nitrogen waste products, etc. to and from cells in the body to help fight diseases and help stabilize body temperature and pH to maintain homeostasis. This system may be seen strictly as a blood distribution network, but some consider the circulatory system as composed of the cardiovascular system, which distributes blood, and the lymphatic system, which distributes lymph. While humans, as well as other vertebrates, have a closed cardiovascular system (meaning that the blood never leaves the network of arteries, veins and capillaries), some invertebrate groups have an open cardiovascular system. The most primitive animal phyla lack circulatory system. The lymphatic system, on the other hand, is an open system.

The main components of the human circulatory system are the heart, the blood, and the blood vessels. The circulatory system includes: the pulmonary circulation, a "loop" through the lungs where blood is oxygenated; and the systemic circulation, a "loop" through the rest of the body to provide oxygenated blood. An average adult contains five to six quarts (roughly 4.7 to 5.7 liters) of blood, which consists of plasma, red blood cells, white blood cells, and platelets. Also, the digestive system works with the circulatory system to provide the

Circulatory System

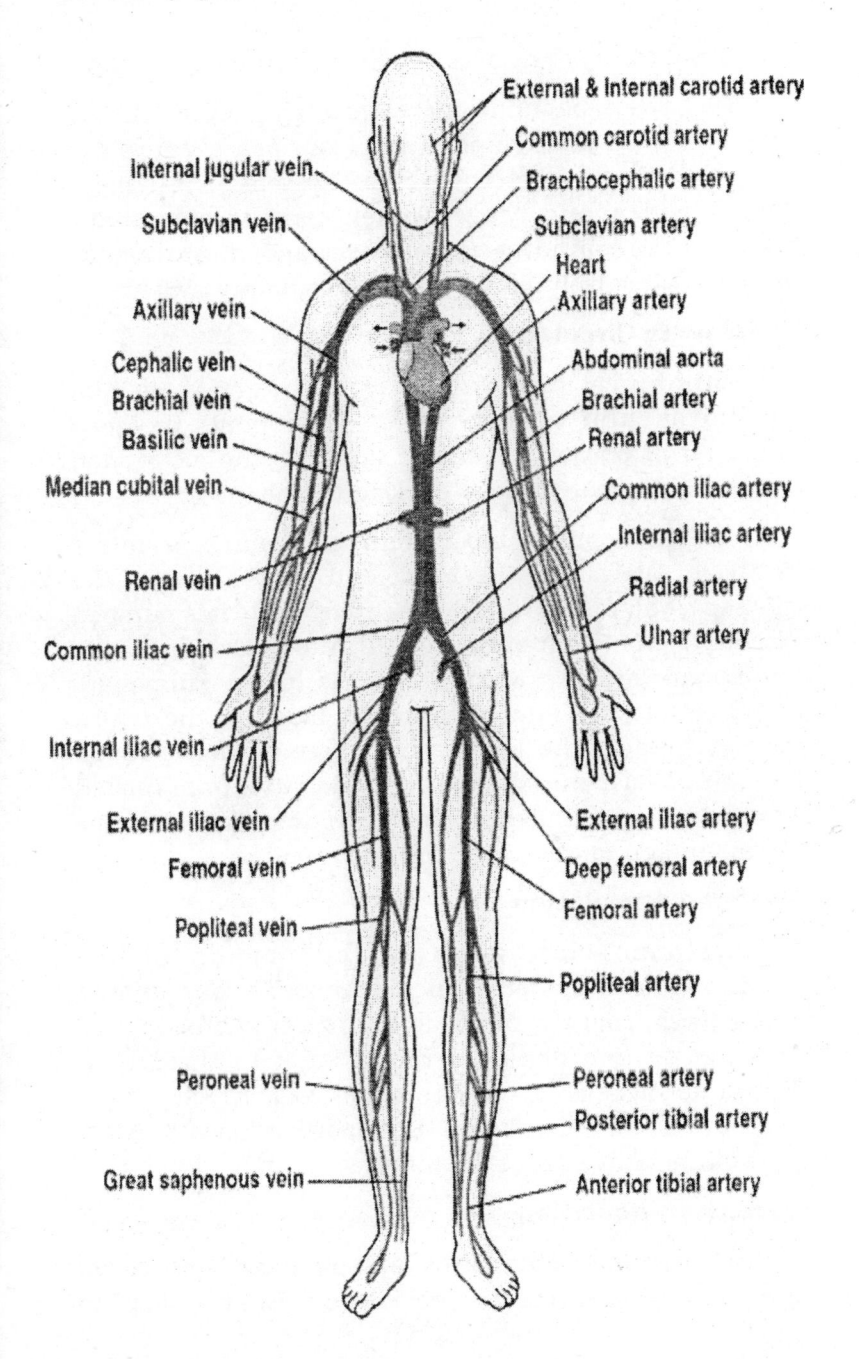

113

nutrients the system needs to keep the heart pumping.

Two types of fluids move through the circulatory system: blood and lymph. The blood, heart, and blood vessels form the cardiovascular system. The lymph, lymph nodes, and lymph vessels form the lymphatic system. The cardiovascular system and the lymphatic system collectively make up the circulatory system.

Pulmonary Circulation

Pulmonary circulation is the portion of the cardiovascular system which transports oxygen-depleted blood away from the heart, to the lungs, and returns oxygenated blood back to the heart.

Oxygen deprived blood from the vena cava enters the right atrium of the heart and flows through the tricuspid valve into the right ventricle where it is pumped through the pulmonary semilunar valve into the pulmonary arteries which go to the lungs. Pulmonary veins return the now oxygen-rich blood to the heart, where it enters the left atrium before flowing through the mitral valve into the left ventricle. Also, from the left ventricle the oxygen-rich blood is pumped out via the aorta, and on to the rest of the body.

Systemic Circulation

Systemic circulation is the portion of the cardiovascular system which transports oxygenated blood away from the heart, to the rest of the body, and returns oxygen-depleted blood back to the heart. Systemic circulation is, distance-wise, much longer than pulmonary circulation, transporting blood to every part of the body except the lungs.

Coronary Circulation

The coronary circulatory system provides a blood supply to the heart. As it provides oxygenated blood to

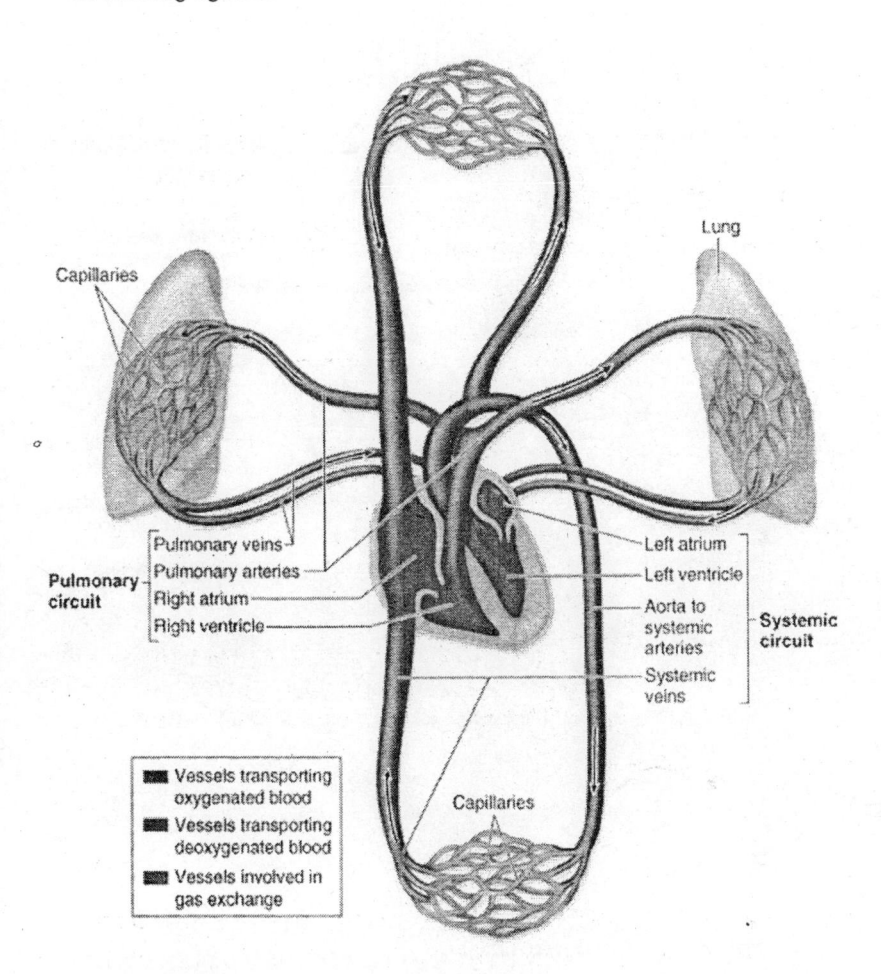

Circulatory System

Diagram labels:
- Lung
- Capillaries
- Pulmonary circuit: Pulmonary veins, Pulmonary arteries, Right atrium, Right ventricle
- Left atrium
- Left ventricle
- Aorta to systemic arteries
- Systemic veins
- Systemic circuit
- Capillaries
- Vessels transporting oxygenated blood
- Vessels transporting deoxygenated blood
- Vessels involved in gas exchange

the heart, it is by definition a part of the systemic circulatory system.

Heart

View from the front, which means the right side of the heart is on the left of the diagram (and vice-versa)Main article: heart

The heart pumps oxygenated blood to the body and deoxygenated blood to the lungs. In the human heart

Exterior structures of the heart

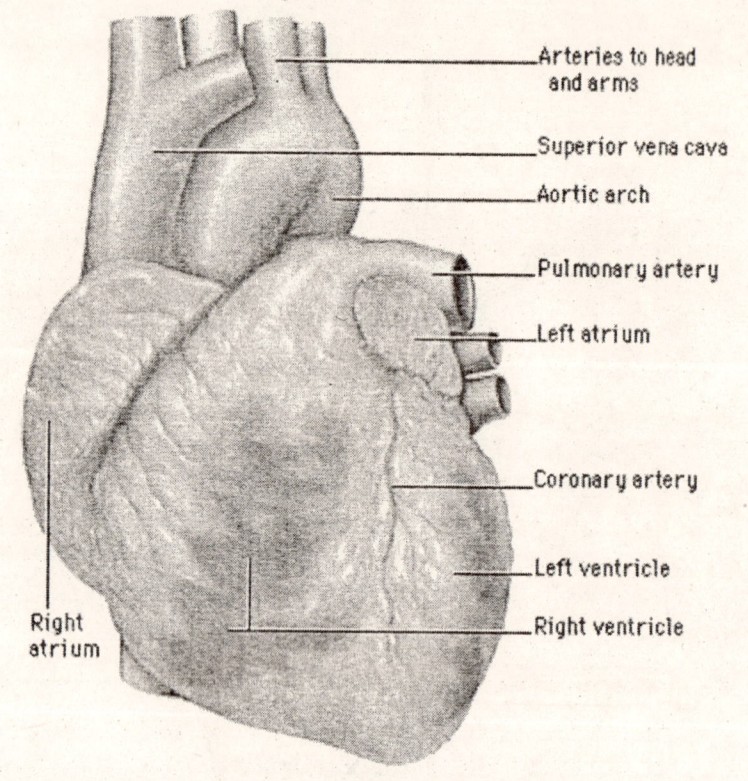

- Arteries to head and arms
- Superior vena cava
- Aortic arch
- Pulmonary artery
- Left atrium
- Coronary artery
- Left ventricle
- Right ventricle
- Right atrium

there is one atrium and one ventricle for each circulation, and with both a systemic and a pulmonary circulation there are four chambers in total: left atrium, left ventricle, right atrium and right ventricle. The right Atrium, which is the upper chamber of the right side. The blood that is returned to the right atrium is deoxygenated (poor in oxygen) and passed into the right ventricle to be pumped through the pulmonary artery to the lungs for re-oxygenation and removal of carbon dioxide. The left atrium receives newly oxygenated blood from the lungs as well as the pulmonary vein which is passed into the strong left ventricle to be pumped through the aorta to the tissues of the body.

Closed Cardiovascular System

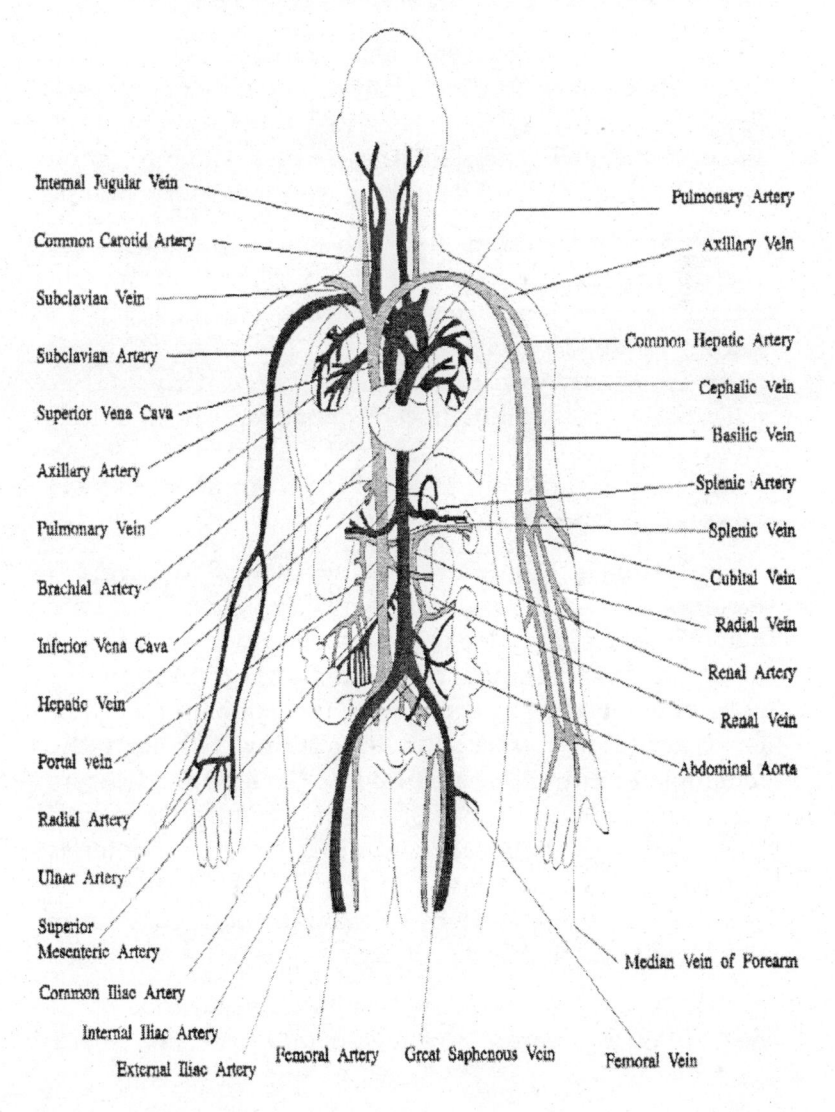

The cardiovascular systems of humans are closed, meaning that the blood never leaves the system. In contrast, oxygen and nutrients diffuse across the blood vessel layers and enters interstitial fluid, which carries oxygen and nutrients to the target cells, and carbon dioxide and wastes in the opposite direction. The other component of the circulatory system, the lymphatic system, is not closed.

Other Vertebrates

The circulatory systems of all vertebrates, as well as of annelids (for example, earthworms) and cephalopods (squid and octopus) are closed, just as in humans. Still, the systems of fish, amphibians, reptiles, and birds show various stages of the evolution of the circulatory system.

In fish, the system has only one circuit, with the blood being pumped through the capillaries of the gills and on to the capillaries of the body tissues. This is known as single cycle circulation. The heart of fish is therefore only a single pump (consisting of two chambers). In amphibians and most reptiles, a double circulatory system is used, but the heart is not always completely separated into two pumps. Amphibians have a three-chambered heart.

In reptiles, the ventricular septum of the heart is incomplete and the pulmonary artery is equipped with a sphincter muscle. This allows a second possible route of blood flow. Instead of blood flowing through the pulmonary artery to the lungs, the sphincter may be contracted to divert this blood flow through the incomplete ventricular septum into the left ventricle and out through the aorta. This means the blood flows from the capillaries to the heart and back to the capillaries instead of to the lungs. This process is useful to ectothermic (cold-blooded) animals in the regulation of their body temperature.

Birds and mammals show complete separation of the heart into two pumps, for a total of four heart chambers;

it is thought that the four-chambered heart of birds evolved independently from that of mammals.

Open Circulatory System

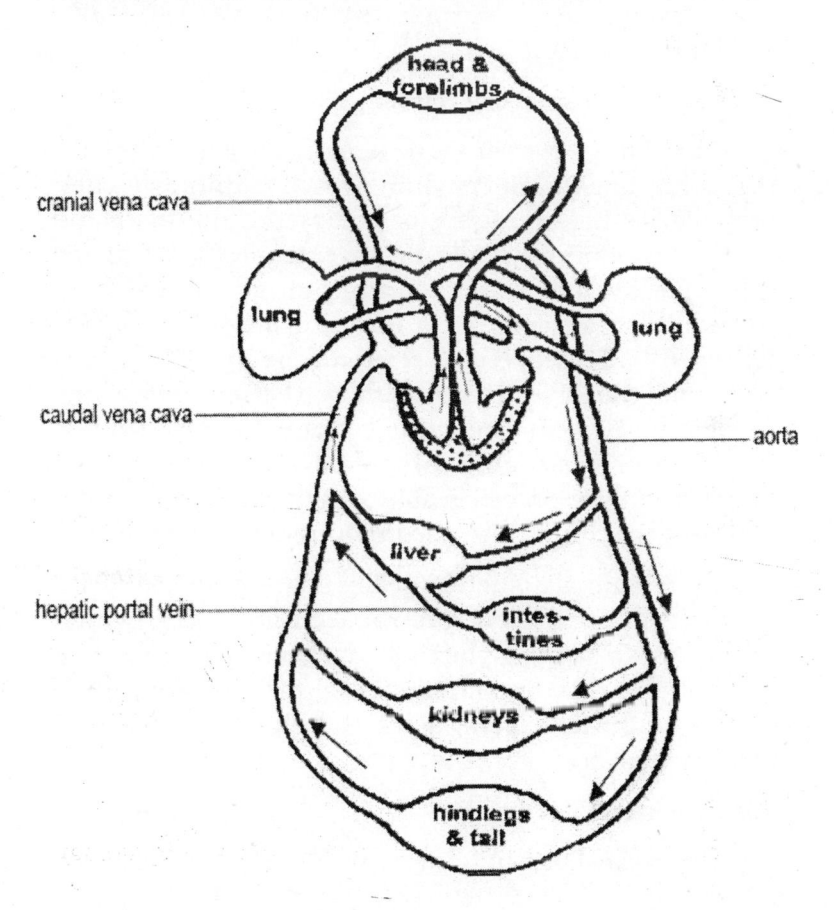

The Open Circulatory System is a system in which fluid (called hemolymph) in a cavity called the hemocoel bathes the organs directly with oxygen and nutrients and there is no distinction between blood and interstitial fluid; this combined fluid is called hemolymph or haemolymph. Muscular movements by the animal during locomotion can facilitate hemolymph movement, but diverting flow from one area to another is limited. When the heart relaxes, blood is drawn back toward the heart through open-ended pores (ostia).

Hemolymph fills all of the interior hemocoel of the body and surrounds all cells. Hemolymph is composed of water, inorganic salts (mostly Na^+, Cl^-, K^+, Mg^{2+}, and Ca^{2+}), and organic compounds (mostly carbohydrates, proteins, and lipids). The primary oxygen transporter molecule is hemocyanin.

There are free-floating cells, the hemocytes, within the hemolymph. They play a role in the arthropod immune system.

Absence of Circulatory System

Circulatory systems are absent in some animals, including flatworms (phylum Platyhelminthes). Their body cavity has no lining or enclosed fluid. Instead a muscular pharynx leads to an extensively branched digestive system that facilitates direct diffusion of nutrients to all cells. The flatworm's dorso-ventrally flattened body shape also restricts the distance of any cell from the digestive system or the exterior of the organism. Oxygen can diffuse from the surrounding water into the cells, and carbon dioxide can diffuse out. Consequently every cell is able to obtain nutrients, water and oxygen without the need of a transport system.

Some animals, such as jellies, have more extensive branching from their gastrovascular cavity (which functions as both a place of digestion and a form of circulation), this branching allows for bodily fluids to reach the outter layers, since the digestion begins in the inner layers.

Measurement Techniques

Electrocardiogram — for cardiac electrophysiology

Sphygmomanometer and stethoscope — for blood pressure

Pulse meter — for cardiac function (heart rate, rhythm, dropped beats)

Pulse — commonly used to determine the heart rate in absence of certain cardiac pathologies

Heart rate variability -- used to measure variations of time intervals between heart beats

Nail bed blanching test — test for perfusion

Vessel cannula or catheter pressure measurement — pulmonary wedge pressure or in older animal experiments.

Health and Disease

Cardiovascular Disease

Congenital Heart Defect

Oxygen Transportation

About 98.5% of the oxygen in a sample of arterial blood in a healthy human breathing air at sea-level pressure is chemically combined with haemoglobin molecules. About 1.5% is physically dissolved in the other blood liquids and not connected to Hgb. The haemoglobin molecule is the primary transporter of oxygen in mammals and many other species.

History of Discovery

The earliest known writings on the circulatory system are found in the Ebers Papyrus (16th century BCE), an ancient Egyptian medical papyrus containing over 700 prescriptions and remedies, both physical and spiritual. In the papyrus, it acknowledges the connection of the heart to the arteries. The Egyptians thought air came in through the mouth and into the lungs and heart. From the heart, the air traveled to every member through the arteries. Although this concept of the circulatory system is greatly flawed, it represents one of the earliest accounts of scientific thought.

The knowledge of circulation of vital fluids through the body was known to Sushruta (6th century BCE). He also seems to have possessed knowledge of the arteries, described as 'channels' by Dwivedi & Dwivedi (2007). The valves of the heart were discovered by a physician of the Hippocratean school around the 4th century BC. However their function was not properly understood then. Because blood pools in the veins after death, arteries look empty. Ancient anatomists assumed they were filled with air and that they were for transport of air.

Greek physician Herophilus distinguished veins from arteries but thought that the pulse was a property of arteries themselves. Greek anatomist Erasistratus observed that arteries that were cut during life bleed. He ascribed the fact to the phenomenon that air escaping from an artery is replaced with blood that entered by very small vessels between veins and arteries. Thus he apparently postulated capillaries but with reversed flow of blood.

The 2nd century AD, Greek physician, Galen, knew that blood vessels carried blood and identified venous (dark red) and arterial (brighter and thinner) blood, each with distinct and separate functions. Growth and energy were derived from venous blood created in the liver from chyle, while arterial blood gave vitality by containing pneuma (air) and originated in the heart. Blood flowed from both creating organs to all parts of the body where it was consumed and there was no return of blood to the heart or liver. The heart did not pump blood around, the heart's motion sucked blood in during diastole and the blood moved by the pulsation of the arteries themselves.

Galen believed that the arterial blood was created by venous blood passing from the left ventricle to the right by passing through 'pores' in the interventricular septum, air passed from the lungs via the pulmonary artery to the left side of the heart. As the arterial blood was created 'sooty' vapors were created and passed to the lungs also via the pulmonary artery to be exhaled.

In 1242, the Arabian physician, Ibn al-Nafis, became the first person to accurately describe the process of pulmonary circulation, for which he is sometimes considered the father of circulatory physiology. Ibn al-Nafis stated in his Commentary on Anatomy in Avicenna's Canon:

"...the blood from the right chamber of the heart must arrive at the left chamber but there is no direct pathway between them. The thick septum of the heart is not perforated and does not have visible pores as some people thought or invisible pores as Galen thought. The blood from the right chamber must flow through the vena arteriosa (pulmonary artery) to the lungs, spread through its substances, be mingled there with air, pass through the arteria venosa (pulmonary vein) to reach the left chamber of the heart and there form the vital spirit..."

Finally William Harvey, a pupil of Hieronymus Fabricius (who had earlier described the valves of the veins without recognizing their function), performed a sequence of experiments, and published Exercitatio Anatomica de Motu Cordis et Sanguinis in Animalibus in 1628, which "demonstrated that there had to be a direct connection between the venous and arterial systems throughout the body, and not just the lungs. Most importantly, he argued that the beat of the heart produced a continuous circulation of blood through minute connections at the extremities of the body. This is is a conceptual leap that was quite different from Ibn al-Nafis' refinement of the anatomy and bloodflow in the heart and lungs." This work, with its essentially correct exposition, slowly convinced the medical world. However, Harvey was not able to identify the capillary system connecting arteries and veins; these were later described by Marcello Malpighi.

7

Respiratory System

A respiratory system's function is to allow gas exchange. The space between the alveoli and the capillaries, the anatomy or structure of the exchange system, and the precise physiological uses of the exchanged gases vary depending on the organism. In humans and other mammals, for example, the anatomical features of the respiratory system include airways, lungs, and the respiratory muscles. Molecules

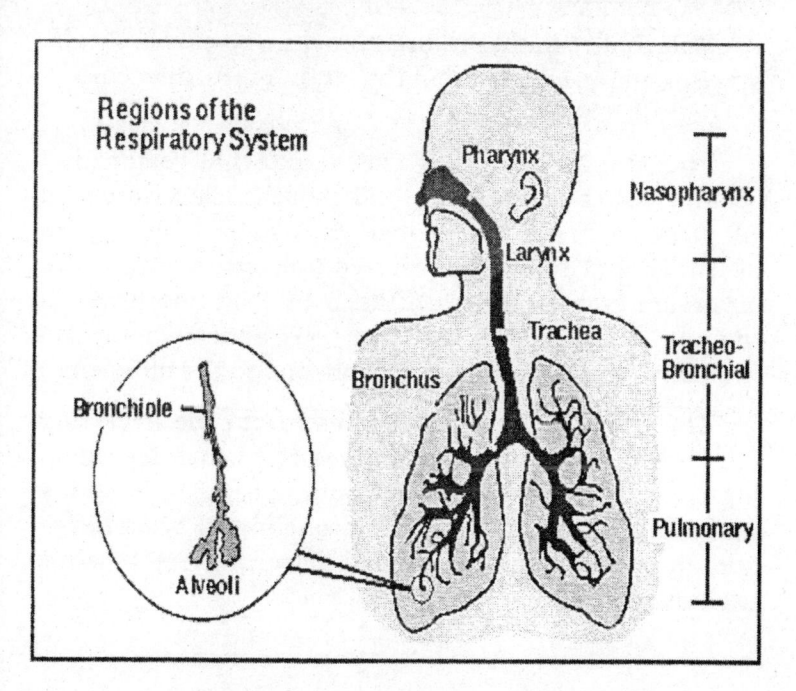

Regions of the Respiratory System

- Pharynx
- Larynx
- Trachea
- Bronchus
- Bronchiole
- Alveoli

- Nasopharynx
- Tracheo-Bronchial
- Pulmonary

of oxygen and carbon dioxide are passively exchanged, by diffusion, between the gaseous external environment and the blood. This exchange process occurs in the alveolar region of the lungs.

Other animals, such as insects, have respiratory systems with very simple anatomical features, and in amphibians even the skin plays a vital role in gas exchange. Plants also have respiratory systems but the directionality of gas exchange can be opposite to that in animals. The respiratory system in plants also includes anatomical features such as holes on the undersides of leaves known as stomata.

The word respiration describes two processes.

Internal or cellular respiration is the process by which glucose or other small molecules are oxidised to produce energy: this requires oxygen and generates carbon dioxide.

External respiration (breathing) involves simply the stage of taking oxygen from the air and returning carbon dioxide to it.

The respiratory tract, where external respiration occurs, starts at the nose and mouth. (Description of respiratory tract from nose to trachea here from overheads) (There is a brief complication where the airstream crosses the path taken by food and drink in the pharynx: air flows on down the trachea where food normally passes down the oesophagus to the stomach.)

The trachea (windpipe) extends from the neck into the thorax, where it divides into right and left main bronchi, which enter the right and left lungs, breaking up as they do so into smaller bronchi and bronchioles and ending in small air sacs or alveoli, where gaseous exchange occurs.

Respiratory System

The lungs are divided first into right and left, the left being smaller to accommodate the heart, then into lobes (three on the right, two on the left) supplied by lobar bronchi.

Bronchi, pulmonary arteries and veins (which supply deoxygenated blood and remove oxygenated blood), bronchial arteries and veins (which supply oxygenated blood to the substance of the lung itself) and lymphatics all enter and leave the lung by its root (or hilum). Lymph nodes blackened by soot particles can often be seen here and the substance of the lung itself may be blackened by soot in city dwellers or heavy smokers.

Each lobe of the lung is further divided into a pyramidal bronchopulmonary segments. Bronchopulmonary segments have the apex of the pyramid in the hilum whence they receive a tertiary bronchus, and appropriate blood vessels. The 10 segments of the right lung and eight of the left are virtually self contained units not in communication with other parts of the lung. This is of obvious use in surgery when appropriate knowledge will allow a practically bloodless excision of a diseased segment.

Gaseous exchange relies on simple diffusion. In order to provide sufficient oxygen and to get rid of sufficient carbon dioxide there must be

- a large surface area for gaseous exchange
- a very short diffusion path between alveolar air and blood
- concentration gradients for oxygen and carbon dioxide between alveolar air and blood.

The surface available in an adult is around 140m2 in an adult, around the area of a singles tennis court. The blood in the alveolar capillaries is separated from

alveolar air by 0.6* in many places (1* = one thousandth of a mm). Diffusion gradients are maintained by
- ventilation (breathing) which renews alveolar air, maintaining oxygen concentration near that of atmospheric air and preventing the accumulation of carbon dioxide
- the flow of blood in alveolar capillaries which continually brings blood with low oxygen concentration and high carbon dioxide concentration

Haemoglobin in blood continually removes dissolved oxygen from the blood and binds with it. The presence of this tennis court, separated from the outside air by a very narrow barrier imposes demands on the respiratory tract.

Outside air:
- varies in temperature. At the alveolar surface it must be at body temperature
- varies from very dry to very humid. At the alveolar surface it must be saturated with water vapour
- contains dust and debris. These must not reach the alveolar wall
- contains micro-organisms, which must be filtered out of the inspired air and disposed of before they reach the alveoli, enter the blood and cause possible problems.

It is easy to see that the temperature and humidity of inspired air will increase as it passes down a long series of tubes lined with a moist mucosa at body temperature. The mechanisms for filtering are not so obvious.

Mucus

The respiratory tract, from nasal cavities to the

smallest bronchi, is lined by a layer of sticky mucus, secreted by the epithelium assisted by small ducted glands. Particles which hit the side wall of the tract are trapped in this mucus. This is encouraged by: (a) the air stream changing direction, as it repeatedly does in a continually dividing tube. (b) random (Brownian) movement of small particles suspended in the airstream.

The first of these works particularly well on more massive particles, the second on smaller bits

Cilia

Once the particles have been sidelined by the mucus they have to be removed, as indeed does the mucous. This is carried out by cilia on the epithelial cells which move the mucous continually up or down the tract towards the nose and mouth. (Those in the nose beat downwards, those in the trachea and below upwards).

The mucus and its trapped particles are and bacteria are then swallowed, taking them to the sterilising vat of the stomach.

Length

The length of the respiratory tract helps in both bringing the air to the right temperature and humidity but hinders the actual ventilation, as a long tract has a greater volume of air trapped within it, and demands a large breath to clear out residual air.

Protection

The entry of food and drink into the larynx is prevented by the structure of the larynx and by the complicated act of swallowing. The larynx is protected by three pairs of folds which close off the airway. In man these have a secondary function, they vibrate in the airstream to produce sounds, the basis of speech and singing. Below the larynx the trachea is usually patent i.e. open, and kept so by rings of cartilage in its walls. However it may be necessary to ensure that this condition is maintained by passing a tube (endotracheal intubation) to maintain the airway, especially post operatively if the patient has been given a muscle relaxant. Another common surgical procedure, tracheotomy, involves a small transverse cut in the neck. If this is done with anatomical knowledge no major structure is disturbed and the opening may be used for a suction tube, a ventilator, or in cases of tracheal obstruction as a permanent airway.

Ventilation and Perfusion

The gills of fish and the lungs of birds allow water and air receptively to flow continually over the exchanging surface. In common with all mammals humans ventilate their lungs by breathing in and out. This reciprocal movement of air is less efficient and is achieved by alternately increasing and decreasing the volume of the chest in breathing. The body's requirements for oxygen vary widely with muscular activity. In violent exercise the rate and depth of ventilation increase greatly: this will only work in conjunction with increase in blood flow, controlled mainly by the rich innervation of the lungs.. Gas exchange can be improved by breathing enriched air, which produces significantly reduced times for track events. Inadequate gas exchange is common in many diseases, producing respiratory distress.

Mechanism of Breathing

In order to grasp the way in which we breathe we have to grasp the following facts:

Each lung is surrounded by a pleural cavity or sac, except where the plumbing joins it to the rest of the body, rather like a hand in a boxing glove. The glove has an

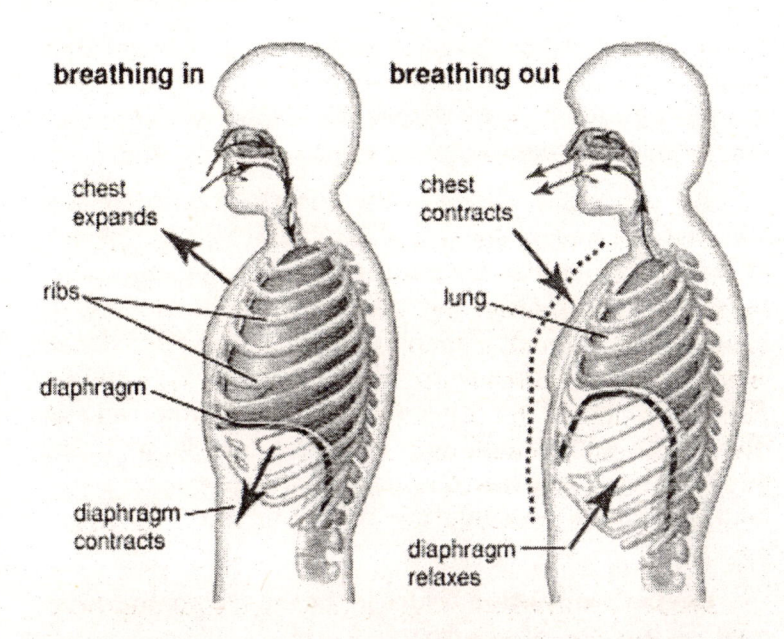

Respiratory System

breathing in
- chest expands
- ribs
- diaphragm
- diaphragm contracts

breathing out
- chest contracts
- lung
- diaphragm relaxes

outer and inner surface, separated by a layer of padding. The pleura, similarly, has two surfaces, but the padding is replaced by a thin layer of fluid.

Each lung is enclosed in a cage bounded below by the diaphragm and at the sides by the chest wall and the mediastinum (technical term for the bit around the heart). It is not usually appreciated that the lung extends so high into the neck. A syringe inserted above a clavicle may pierce the lung.

Breathing works by making the cage bigger: the pleural layers slide over each other and the pressure in the lung is decreased, so air is sucked in. Breathing out does the reverse, the cage collapses and air is expelled. The main component acting here is the diaphragm. This is a layer of muscle which is convex above, domed, and squashed in the centre by the heart. When it contracts it flattens and increases the space above it. When it relaxes the abdominal contents push it up again. The proportion of breathing which is diaphragmatic varies from person to person. For instance breathing in children and pregnant women is largely diaphragmatic, and there is said to be more diaphragmatic respiration in women than in men.

The process is helped by the ribs which move up and out also increasing the space available. The complexity of breathing increases as does the need for efficiency. In **quiet respiration**, say whilst lying on ones back, almost all movement is diaphragmatic and the chest wall is still. This will increase thoracic volume by 500-700ml. The expansion of the lung deforms the flexible walls of the alveoli and bronchi and stretches the elastic fibres in the lung. When the diaphragm relaxes elastic recoil and abdominal musculature reposition the diaphragm again.

Deeper respiration brings in the muscles of the chest wall, so that the ribs move too.

We must therefore understand the skeleton and muscular system of the thoracic wall.

The 12 pairs of ribs pass around the thoracic wall, articulating via synovial joints with the vertebral column - in fact two per rib. The ribs then curve outwards then forwards and downwards and attach to the sternum via the flexible costal cartilages. The first seven pairs of ribs (true ribs) attach directly, the next five hitch a lift on each other and the last two float i.e. are unattached. Costal cartilages are flexible. The first rib is rather different, short, flattened above and below and suspended beneath a set of fairly hefty muscles passing up into the neck, the scalene muscles. Between the ribs run two sets of intercostal muscles, the external intercostals running forward and downwards, the internal intercostals running up and back. These two muscle sheets thus run between ribs with fibres roughly at right angles. When they contract each rib moves closer to its neighbours. Because the lowest ribs float, and the first rib is suspended from the scalene muscles contraction of the intercostal muscles tends to lift rib two towards rib 1, and so on. The ribs are all, therefore pulled up towards the horizontal, increasing anteroomposterior and lateral thoracic diameters.

These movements are sometimes divided intopump handle movements, the rib abducting on its vertebral joints and bucket handle movements, the rib rotating on its axis around anterior and posterior attachments: these are not necessarily helpful.

With more and more effort put into deeper and deeper breathing the scalene muscles of the neck contract, raising the first rib and hence the rest of the cage, then other neck muscles and even those of the upper limb become involved. A patient with difficulty in breathing often grips a table edge in order to stabilise the limbs so that their muscles can be used to help in moving the thoracic wall.

Problems

The lungs sometimes fail to maintain an adequate supply of air. The earliest cases of this are seen in infant respiratory distress syndrome. In premature infants (less than about 2 lbs or 37 weeks the cells which make surfactant are not yet active. Surfactant reduces the surface tension in the fluid on the surface of the alveoli, allowing them to expand at the first breath, and remain open thereafter. The sacs either fail to expand, or expand then collapse on expiration and result in laboured breathing. In adults a similar syndrome is due to accidental inhalation of water, smoke, vomit or chemical fumes.

Acute bronchitis is due to infection of the bronchial tree, which may have impaired function due to fluid accumulation. Pneumonia involves the lung proper.

Lung cancers a malignancy that may spread to other tissues via the lymphatics in the lung roots.

The respiratory system can be divided into 3 regions:

- Nasopharynx Region: the head region, including the nose, mouth, pharynx, and larynx
- Tracheobronchial Region: includes the trachea, bronchi, and bronchioles
- Pulmonary (Alveolar) Region: comprised of the alveoli; the exchange of oxygen and carbon dioxide through the process of respiration occurs in the alveolar region.

The Design of the Respiratory System

The human gas exchanging organ, the lung, is located in the thorax, where its delicate tissues are protected by the bony and muscular thoracic cage. The lung provides the organism with a continuous flow of oxygen and clears the blood of the gaseous waste product, carbon dioxide. Atmospheric air is pumped in and out regularly through a system of pipes, called conducting airways, which join the gas exchange region with the outside of the body. The airways can be divided into upper and lower airway systems. The transition between the two systems is located where the pathways of the respiratory and digestive systems cross, just at the top of the larynx.

The upper airway system comprises the nose and the paranasal cavities, called sinuses, the pharynx, or throat, and partly also the oral cavity, since it may be used for breathing. The lower airway system consists of the larynx, the trachea, the stem bronchi, and all the airways ramifying intensively within the lungs, such as the intrapulmonary bronchi, the bronchioles, and the alveolar ducts. For respiration, the collaboration of other organ systems is clearly essential. The diaphragm, as the main respiratory muscle, and the intercostal muscles of the chest wall play an essential role by generating, under the control of the central nervous system, the pumping action on the lung. The muscles expand and contract the internal space of the thorax, whose bony framework is formed by the ribs and the thoracic vertebrae. The contribution of the lung and chest wall (ribs and muscles) to respiration is described below in The mechanics of breathing. The blood, as a carrier for the gases, and the circulatory system (i.e., the heart and the blood vessels) are mandatory elements of a working respiratory system.

The design of the respiratory system » Morphology of the upper airways. The nose

The nose is the external protuberance of an internal space, the nasal cavity. It is subdivided into a left and right canal by a thin medial cartilaginous and bony wall, the nasal septum. Each canal opens to the face by a nostril and into the pharynx by the choana. The floor of the nasal cavity is formed by the palate, which also forms the roof of the oral cavity. The complex shape of the nasal cavity is due to projections of bony ridges, the superior, middle, and inferior turbinate bones (or conchae), from the lateral wall. The passageways thus formed below each ridge are called the superior, middle, and inferior nasal meatuses.

On each side, the intranasal space communicates with a series of neighbouring air-filled cavities within the skull (the paranasal sinuses) and also, via the nasolacrimal duct, with the lacrimal apparatus in the corner of the eye. The duct drains the lacrimal fluid into the nasal cavity. This fact explains why nasal respiration can be rapidly impaired or even impeded during weeping: the lacrimal fluid is not only overflowing into tears, it is also flooding the nasal cavity.

The paranasal sinuses are sets of paired single or multiple cavities of variable size. Most of their development takes place after birth, and they reach their final size toward the age of 20 years. The sinuses are located in four different skull bones—the maxilla, the frontal, the ethmoid, and the sphenoid bones. Correspondingly, they are called the maxillary sinus, which is the largest cavity; the frontal sinus; the ethmoid sinuses; and the sphenoid sinus, which is located in the upper posterior wall of the nasal cavity. The sinuses have two principal functions: because they are filled with air, they help keep the weight of the skull within reasonable limits, and they serve as resonance chambers for the human voice.

The nasal cavity with its adjacent spaces is lined by a respiratory mucosa. Typically, the mucosa of the nose contains mucus-secreting glands and venous plexuses; its top cell layer, the epithelium, consists principally of two cell types, ciliated and secreting cells. This structural design reflects the particular ancillary functions of the nose and of the upper airways in general with respect to respiration. They clean, moisten, and warm the inspired air, preparing it for intimate contact with the delicate tissues of the gas-exchange area. During expiration through the nose, the air is dried and cooled, a process that saves water and energy.

Two regions of the nasal cavity have a different lining. The vestibule, at the entrance of the nose, is lined by skin that bears short thick hairs called vibrissae. In the roof of the nose, the olfactory organ with its sensory epithelium checks the quality of the inspired air. About two dozen olfactory nerves convey the sensation of smell from the olfactory cells through the bony roof of the nasal cavity to the central nervous system.

Respiratory System

The Pharynx

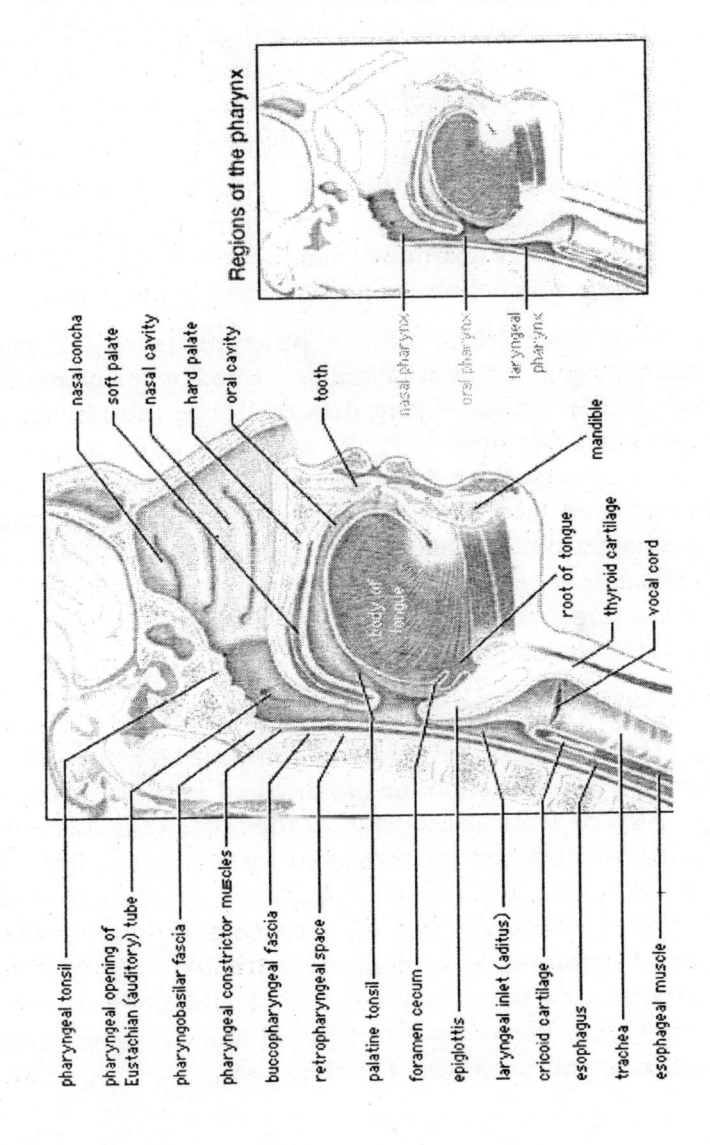

For the anatomical description, the pharynx can be divided into three floors. The upper floor, the nasopharynx, is primarily a passageway for air and secretions from the nose to the oral pharynx. It is also connected to the tympanic cavity of the middle ear through the auditory tubes that open on both lateral walls. The act of swallowing opens briefly the normally collapsed auditory tubes and allows the middle ears to be aerated and pressure differences to be equalized. In the posterior wall of the nasopharynx is located a lymphatic organ, the pharyngeal tonsil. When it is enlarged (as in tonsil hypertrophy or adenoid vegetation), it may interfere with nasal respiration and alter the resonance pattern of the voice.

The middle floor of the pharynx connects anteriorly to the mouth and is therefore called the oral pharynx or oropharynx. It is delimited from the nasopharynx by the soft palate, which roofs the posterior part of the oral cavity.

The lower floor of the pharynx is called the hypopharynx. Its anterior wall is formed by the posterior part of the tongue. Lying directly above the larynx, it represents the site where the pathways of air and food cross each other: Air from the nasal cavity flows into the larynx, and food from the oral cavity is routed to the esophagus directly behind the larynx. The epiglottis, a cartilaginous, leaf-shaped flap, functions as a lid to the larynx and, during the act of swallowing, controls the traffic of air and food.

The Larynx

The larynx is an organ of complex structure that serves a dual function: as an air canal to the lungs and a controller of its access, and as the organ of phonation. Sound is produced by forcing air through a sagittal slit formed by the vocal cords, the glottis. This causes not only the vocal cords but also the column of air above them to vibrate. As evidenced by trained singers, this function can be closely controlled and finely tuned. Control is achieved by a number of muscles innervated by the laryngeal nerves. For the precise function of the

Respiratory System

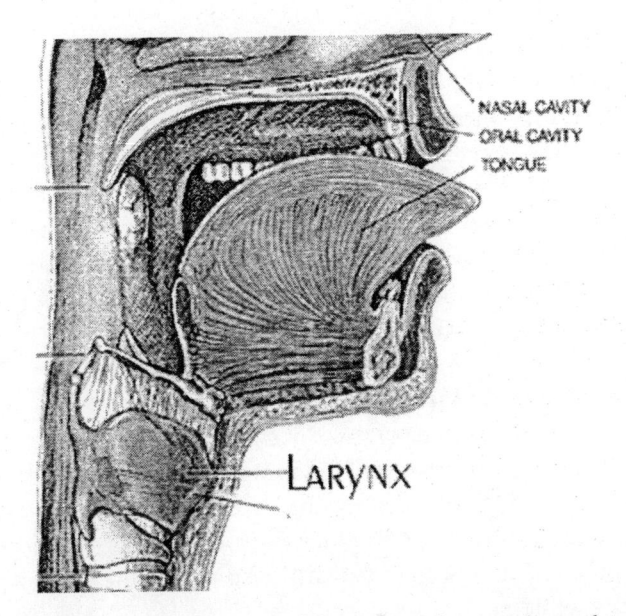

muscular apparatus, the muscles must be anchored to a stabilizing framework. The laryngeal skeleton consists of almost a dozen pieces of cartilage, most of them very small, interconnected by ligaments and membranes. The largest cartilage of the larynx, the thyroid cartilage, is made of two plates fused anteriorly in the midline. At the upper end of the fusion line is an incision, the thyroid notch; below it is a forward projection, the laryngeal prominence. Both of these structures are easily felt through the skin. The angle between the two cartilage plates is sharper and the prominence more marked in men than in women, which has given this structure the common name of Adam's apple. Behind the shieldlike thyroid cartilage, the vocal cords span the laryngeal lumen. They correspond to elastic ligaments attached anteriorly in the angle of the thyroid shield and posteriorly to a pair of small pyramidal pieces of cartilage, the arytenoid cartilages. The vocal ligaments are part of a tube, resembling an organ pipe, made of elastic tissue. Just above the vocal cords, the epiglottis is also attached to the back of the thyroid plate by its stalk. The cricoid, another large cartilaginous piece of the laryngeal skeleton, has a signet-ring shape. The broad plate of the ring lies in the posterior wall of the larynx and the narrow arch in the anterior wall. The cricoid is located below the thyroid cartilage, to which it is joined in an articulation reinforced by ligaments. The transverse axis of the joint allows a hingelike rotation between the two cartilages. This movement tilts the cricoid plate with respect to the shield of the thyroid cartilage and hence alters the distance between them. Because the arytenoid cartilages rest upright on the cricoid plate, they follow its tilting movement. This mechanism plays an important role in altering length and tension of the vocal cords. The arytenoid cartilages articulate with the cricoid plate and hence are able to rotate and slide to close and open the glottis.

Viewed frontally, the lumen of the laryngeal tube has an hourglass shape, with its narrowest width at the glottis. Just above the vocal cords there is an additional pair of mucosal folds called the false vocal cords or the vestibular folds. Like the true vocal cords, they are also formed by the free end of a fibroelastic membrane. Between the vestibular folds and the vocal cords, the laryngeal space enlarges and forms lateral pockets extending upward. This space is called the ventricle of the larynx. Because the gap between the vestibular folds is always larger than the gap between the vocal cords, the latter can easily be seen from above with the laryngoscope, an instrument designed for visual inspection of the interior of the larynx.

The muscular apparatus of the larynx comprises two functionally distinct groups. The intrinsic muscles act directly or indirectly on the shape, length, and tension of the vocal cords. The extrinsic muscles act on the larynx as a whole, moving it upward (e.g., during high-pitched phonation or swallowing) or downward. The intrinsic muscles attach to the skeletal components of the larynx itself; the extrinsic muscles join the laryngeal skeleton cranially to the hyoid bone or to the pharynx and caudally to the sternum (breastbone).

The Trachea and the Stem Bronchi

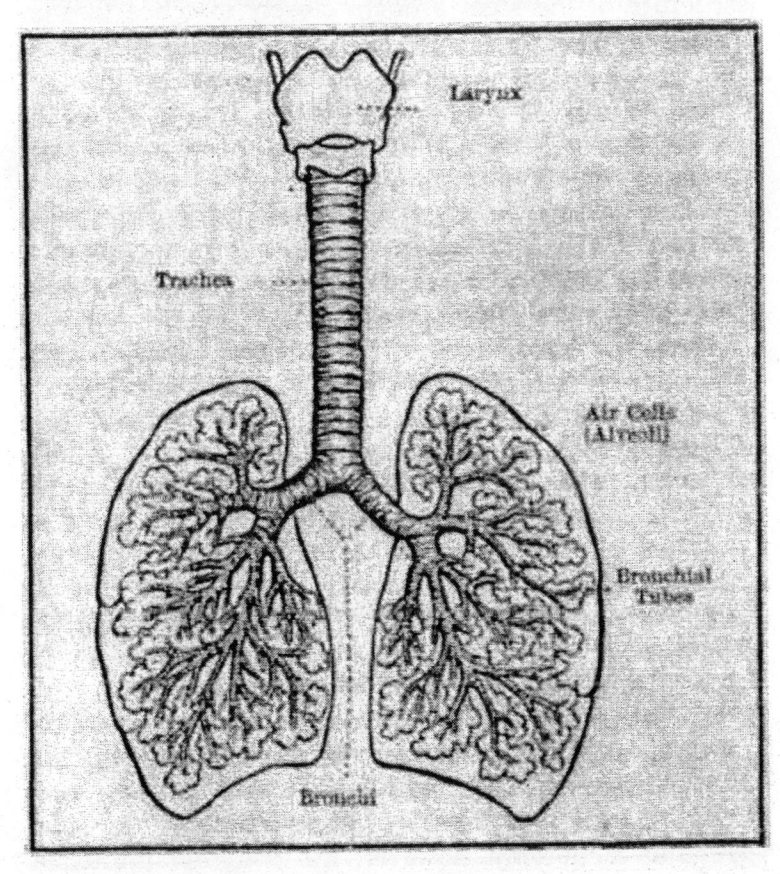

Below the larynx lies the trachea, a tube about 10 to 12 centimetres long and two centimetres wide. Its wall is stiffened by 16 to 20 characteristic horseshoe-shaped, incomplete cartilage rings that open toward the back and are embedded in a dense connective tissue. The dorsal wall contains a strong layer of transverse smooth muscle fibres that spans the gap of the cartilage. The interior of the trachea is lined by the typical respiratory epithelium. The mucosal layer contains mucous glands.

At its lower end, the trachea divides in an inverted Y into the two stem (or main) bronchi, one each for the left and right lung. The right main bronchus has a larger diameter, is oriented more vertically, and is shorter than the left main bronchus. The practical consequence of this arrangement is that foreign bodies passing beyond the larynx will usually slip into the right lung. The structure of the stem bronchi closely matches that of the trachea.

Structural Design of the Airway Tree

The hierarchy of the dividing airways, and partly also of the blood vessels penetrating the lung, largely determines the internal lung structure. Functionally the intrapulmonary airway system can be subdivided into three zones, a proximal, purely conducting zone, a peripheral, purely gas-exchanging zone, and a transitional zone in between, where both functions grade into one another. From a morphological point of view, however, it makes sense to distinguish the relatively thick-walled, purely air-conducting tubes from those branches of the airway tree structurally designed to permit gas exchange.

The structural design of the airway tree is functionally important because the branching pattern plays a role in determining air flow and particle deposition. In modeling the human airway tree, it is generally agreed that the airways branch according to the rules of irregular dichotomy. Regular dichotomy means that each branch of a treelike structure gives rise to two daughter branches of identical dimensions. In irregular dichotomy, however, the daughter branches may differ greatly in length and diameter. The models calculate the average path from the trachea to the lung periphery as consisting of about 24–25 generations of branches. Individual paths, however, may range from 11 to 30 generations. The transition between the conductive and the respiratory portions of an airway lies on average at the end of the 16th generation, if the trachea is counted as generation 0. The conducting airways comprise the trachea, the two stem bronchi, the bronchi, and the bronchioles. Their function is to further warm, moisten, and clean the inspired air and distribute it to the gas-exchanging zone of the lung. They are lined by the typical respiratory epithelium with ciliated cells and numerous interspersed mucus-secreting goblet cells. Ciliated cells are present far down in the airway tree, their height decreasing with the narrowing of the tubes, as does the frequency of goblet cells. In bronchioles the goblet cells are completely replaced by another type of secretory cells named Clara cells. The epithelium is covered by a layer of low-viscosity fluid, within which the cilia exert a synchronized, rhythmic beat directed outward. In larger airways, this fluid layer is topped by a blanket of mucus of high viscosity. The mucus layer is dragged along by the ciliary action and carries the intercepted particles toward the pharynx, where they are swallowed. This design can be compared to a conveyor belt for particles, and indeed the mechanism is referred to as the mucociliary escalator.

The Lungs

The organ lung is parted into two slightly unequal portions, a left lung and a right lung, which occupy most of the intrathoracic space. The space between them is filled by the mediastinum, which corresponds to a connective tissue space containing the heart, major blood vessels, the trachea with the stem bronchi, the esophagus, and the thymus gland. The right lung represents 56 percent of the total lung volume and is composed of three lobes, a superior, middle, and inferior lobe, separated from each other by a deep horizontal and an oblique fissure. The left lung, smaller in volume because of the asymmetrical position of the heart, has only two lobes separated by an oblique fissure. In the thorax, the two lungs rest with their bases on the diaphragm, while their apexes extend above the first rib. Medially, they are connected with the mediastinum at the hilum, a circumscribed area where airways, blood and lymphatic vessels, and nerves enter or leave the lungs. The inside of the thoracic cavities and the lung surface are covered with serous membranes, respectively the parietal pleura and the visceral pleura, which are in direct continuity at the hilum. Depending on the subjacent structures, the parietal pleura can be subdivided into three portions: the mediastinal, costal, and diaphragmatic pleurae. The lung surfaces facing these pleural areas are named accordingly, since the shape of the lungs is determined by the shape of the pleural cavities. Because of the presence of pleural recesses, which form a kind of reserve space, the pleural cavity is larger than the lung volume.

During inspiration, the recesses are partly opened by the expanding lung, thus allowing the lung to increase in volume. Although the hilum is the only place where the lungs are secured to surrounding structures, the lungs are maintained in close apposition to the thoracic wall by a negative pressure between visceral and parietal pleurae. A thin film of extracellular fluid between the pleurae enables the lungs to move smoothly along the walls of the cavity during breathing. If the serous membranes become inflamed (pleurisy), respiratory movements can be painful. If air enters a pleural cavity (pneumothorax), the lung immediately collapses owing to its inherent elastic properties, and breathing is abolished on this side.

Control of Breathing

Breathing is an automatic and rhythmic act produced by networks of neurons in the hindbrain (the pons and medulla). The neural networks direct muscles that form the walls of the thorax and abdomen and produce pressure gradients that move air into and out of the lungs. The respiratory rhythm and the length of each phase of respiration are set by reciprocal stimulatory and inhibitory interconnection of these brain-stem neurons.

An important characteristic of the human respiratory system is its ability to adjust breathing patterns to changes in both the internal milieu and the external environment. Ventilation increases and decreases in proportion to swings in carbon dioxide production and oxygen consumption caused by changes in metabolic rate. The respiratory system is also able to compensate for disturbances that affect the mechanics of breathing, such as the airway narrowing that occurs in an asthmatic attack. Breathing also undergoes appropriate adjustments when the mechanical advantage of the respiratory muscles is altered by postural changes or by movement.

This flexibility in breathing patterns in large part arises from sensors distributed throughout the body that send signals to the respiratory neuronal networks in the brain. Chemoreceptors detect changes in blood oxygen levels and change the acidity of the blood and brain. Mechanoreceptors monitor the expansion of the lung, the size of the airway, the force of respiratory muscle contraction, and the extent of muscle shortening.

Although the diaphragm is the major muscle of

Sinus Cavity

Nose

Throat

Trachea

Three Lobes of Right Lung

Two Lobes of Left Lung

Diaphragm

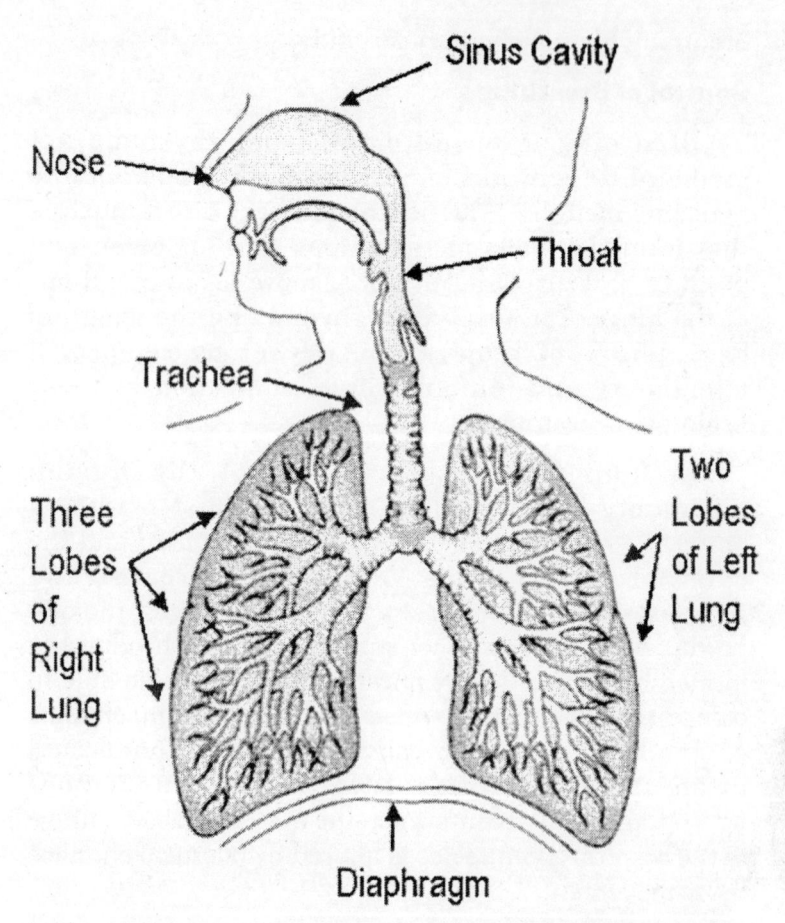

breathing, its respiratory action is assisted and augmented by a complex assembly of other muscle groups. Intercostal muscles inserting on the ribs, the abdominal muscles, and muscles such as the scalene and sternocleidomastoid that attach both to the ribs and to the cervical spine at the base of the skull also play an important role in the exchange of air between the atmosphere and the lungs. In addition, laryngeal muscles and muscles in the oral and nasal pharynx adjust the resistance of movement of gases through the upper airways during both inspiration and expiration.

Although the use of these different muscle groups adds considerably to the flexibility of the breathing act, they also complicate the regulation of breathing. These same muscles are used to perform a number of other functions, such as speaking, chewing and swallowing, and maintaining posture. Perhaps because the "respiratory" muscles are employed in performing nonrespiratory functions, breathing can be influenced by higher brain centres and even controlled voluntarily to a substantial degree. An outstanding example of voluntary control is the ability to suspend breathing by holding one's breath. Input into the respiratory control system from higher brain centres may help optimize breathing so that not only are metabolic demands satisfied by breathing but ventilation also is accomplished with minimal use of energy.

The Mechanics of Breathing

Air moves in and out of the lungs in response to differences in pressure. When the air pressure within the alveolar spaces falls below atmospheric pressure, air enters the lungs (inspiration), provided the larynx is open; when the air pressure within the alveoli exceeds atmospheric pressure, air is blown from the lungs (expiration). The flow of air is rapid or slow in proportion to the magnitude of the pressure difference. Because atmospheric pressure remains relatively constant, flow is determined by how much above or below atmospheric pressure the pressure within the lungs rises or falls.

Alveolar pressure fluctuations are caused by expansion and contraction of the lungs resulting from tensing and relaxing of the muscles of the chest and abdomen. Each small increment of expansion transiently increases the space enclosing lung air. There is, therefore, less air per unit of volume in the lungs and pressure falls. A difference in air pressure between atmosphere and lungs is created, and air flows in until equilibrium with atmospheric pressure is restored at a higher lung volume. When the muscles of inspiration relax, the volume of chest and lungs decreases, lung air becomes transiently compressed, its pressure rises above atmospheric pressure, and flow into the atmosphere results until pressure equilibrium is reached at the original lung volume. This, then, is the sequence of events during each normal respiratory cycle: lung volume change leading to pressure difference, resulting in flow of air into or out of the lung and establishment of a new lung volume.

Gas Exchange

Respiratory gases—oxygen and carbon dioxide—move between the air and the blood across the respiratory exchange surfaces in the lungs. The structure of the human lung provides an immense internal surface that facilitates gas exchange between the alveoli and the blood in the pulmonary capillaries. The area of the alveolar surface in the adult human is about 100 square metres. Gas exchange across the membranous barrier between the alveoli and capillaries is enhanced by the thin nature of the membrane, about 0.5 micrometre, or 1/100 of the diameter of a human hair.

Respiratory gases move between the environment and the respiring tissues by two principal mechanisms, convection and diffusion. Convection, or mass flow, is responsible for movement of air from the environment into the lungs and for movement of blood between the lungs and the tissues. Respiratory gases also move by diffusion across tissue barriers such as membranes. Diffusion is the primary mode of transport of gases between air and blood in the lungs and between blood and respiring tissues in the body. The process of diffusion is driven by the difference in partial pressures of a gas between two locales. In a mixture of gases, the partial pressure of each gas is directly proportional to its concentration. The partial pressure of a gas in fluid is a measure of its tendency to leave the fluid when exposed to a gas or fluid that does not contain that gas. A gas will diffuse from an area of greater partial pressure to an area of lower partial pressure regardless of the distribution of the partial pressures of other gases. There are large changes in the partial pressures of oxygen and carbon dioxide as these gases move between air and the respiring tissues. The partial pressure of carbon dioxide in this pathway is lower than the partial pressure of oxygen, due to differing modes of transport in the blood, but almost equal quantities of the two gases are involved in metabolism and gas exchange.

8

Endocrine and Excretory System

ENDOCRINE SYSTEM

Any of the systems found in animals for the production of hormones, substances that regulate the functioning of the organism. Such a system may range, at its simplest, from the neurosecretory, involving one or more centres in the nervous system, to the complex array of glands found in the human endocrine system.

Group of ductless glands that secrete hormones

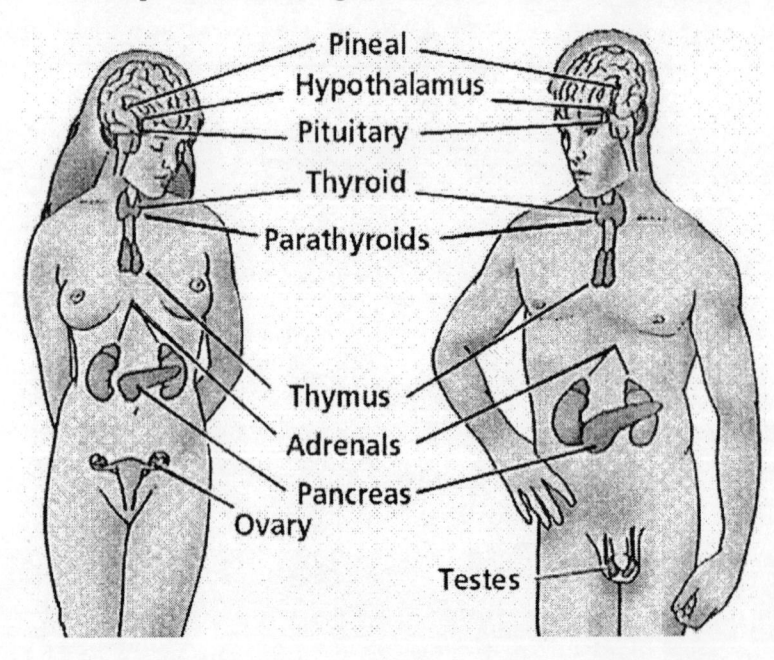

necessary for normal growth and development, reproduction, and homeostasis.

In humans, the major endocrine glands are the hypothalamus, pituitary, pineal, thyroid, parathyroids, adrenals, islets of Langerhans in the pancreas, ovaries, and testes. Secretion is regulated either by regulators in a gland that detect high or low levels of a chemical and inhibit or stimulate secretion or by a complex mechanism involving the hypothalamus and the pituitary. Tumours that produce hormones can throw off this balance. Diseases of the endocrine system result from over- or underproduction of a hormone or from an abnormal response to a hormone.

Group of ductless glands that regulate body processes by secreting chemical substances called hormones. Hormones act on nearby tissues or are carried in the bloodstream to act on specific target organs and distant tissues. Diseases of the endocrine system can result from the oversecretion or undersecretion of hormones or from the inability of target organs or tissues to respond to hormones effectively.

It is important to distinguish between an endocrine gland, which discharges hormones into the bloodstream, and an exocrine gland, which secretes substances through a duct opening in a gland onto an external or internal body surface. Salivary glands and sweat glands are examples of exocrine glands. Both saliva, secreted by the salivary glands, and sweat, secreted by the sweat glands, act on local tissues near the duct openings. In contrast, the hormones secreted by endocrine glands are carried by the circulation to exert their actions on tissues remote from the site of their secretion.

As far back as 3000 bce, the ancient Chinese were able to diagnose and provide effective treatments for some endocrinologic disorders. For example, seaweed, which is rich in iodine, was prescribed for the treatment of goitre (enlargement of the thyroid gland). Perhaps the earliest demonstration of direct endocrinologic intervention in humans was the castration of men who could then be relied upon, more or less, to safeguard the chastity of women living in harems. During the Middle Ages and later, the practice persisting well into the 19th century, prepubertal boys were sometimes castrated to preserve the purity of their treble voices. Castration established the testes (testicles) as the source of substances responsible for the development and maintenance of "maleness."

Function of the Endocrine System—The Nature of Endocrine Regulation

Endocrine gland secretion is not a haphazard process; it is subject to precise, intricate control so that its effects may be integrated with those of the nervous system and the immune system. The simplest level of control over endocrine gland secretion resides at the endocrine gland itself. The signal for an endocrine gland to secrete more or less of its hormone is related to the concentration of some substance, either a hormone that influences the function of the gland (a tropic hormone), a biochemical product (e.g., glucose), or a biologically important element (e.g., calcium or potassium). Because each endocrine gland has a rich supply of blood, each gland is able to detect small changes in the concentrations of its regulating substances.

Some endocrine glands are controlled by a simple negative feedback mechanism. For example, negative feedback signaling mechanisms in the parathyroid glands (located in the neck) rely on the binding activity of calcium-sensitive receptors that are located on the surface of parathyroid cells. Decreased serum calcium concentrations result in decreased calcium receptor binding activity that stimulates the secretion of parathyroid hormone from the parathyroid glands. The increased serum concentration of parathyroid hormone stimulates bone resorption (breakdown) to release calcium into the blood and reabsorption of calcium in the kidney to retain calcium in the blood, thereby restoring serum calcium concentrations to normal levels. In contrast, negative feedback mechanisms are activated by increased serum calcium concentrations, which results in increased calcium receptor-binding activity and inhibition of parathyroid hormone secretion by the parathyroid glands. This allows serum calcium concentrations to decrease to normal levels. Therefore, in people with normal parathyroid glands, serum calcium concentrations are maintained within a very narrow range even in the presence of large changes in calcium intake or excessive losses of calcium from the body.

There are also positive feedback control systems, in which a substance stimulates the secretion of a hormone and the hormone acts to reduce the serum concentrations of the substance. For example, high blood glucose concentrations stimulate insulin secretion from the beta cells of the islets of Langerhans in the pancreas. Insulin stimulates glucose uptake by skeletal muscle and adipose tissue and decreases glucose production by the liver, thereby promoting glucose storage and reducing blood glucose concentrations.

Control of the hormonal secretions of other endocrine glands is more complex, because the glands themselves are target organs of a regulatory system called the hypothalamic-pituitary-target gland axis. The major mechanisms in this regulatory system consist of complex interconnecting negative feedback loops that involve the hypothalamus (a structure located at the base of the brain and above the pituitary gland), the anterior pituitary gland, and the target gland. The hypothalamus produces specific neurohormones that stimulate the pituitary gland to secrete specific pituitary hormones that affect any of a number of target organs, including the adrenal cortex, the gonads (testes and ovaries), and the thyroid gland. Therefore, the hypothalamic-pituitary-target gland axis allows for both neural and hormonal input into hormone production by the target gland.

When stimulated by the appropriate pituitary hormone, the target gland secretes its hormone (target gland hormone) that then combines with receptors located on its target tissues. These receptors include receptors located on the pituitary cells that make the particular hormone that governs the target gland. Should the amount of target gland hormone in the blood increase, the hormone's actions on its target organs increases. In the pituitary gland, the target gland hormone acts to decrease the secretion of the appropriate pituitary hormone, which results in less stimulation of the target gland and a decrease in the production of hormone by the target gland. Conversely, if hormone production by a target gland should decrease, the decrease in serum concentrations of the target gland hormone leads to an increase in secretion of the pituitary hormone in an attempt to restore target gland hormone production to normal. The effect of the target gland hormone on its target tissues is quantitative; that is, within limits, the greater (or lesser) the amount of target gland hormone bound to receptors in the target tissues, the greater (or lesser) the response of the target tissues.

In the hypothalamic-pituitary-target gland axis, a second negative feedback loop is superimposed on the first negative feedback loop. In this second loop, the target gland hormone binds to nerve cells in the hypothalamus, thereby inhibiting the secretion of specific hypothalamic-releasing hormones (neurohormones) that stimulate the secretion of pituitary hormones (an important element in the first negative feedback loop). The hypothalamic neurohormones are released within a set of veins that connects the hypothalamus to the pituitary gland (the hypophyseal-portal circulation), and therefore the neurohormones reach the pituitary gland in high concentrations. Target gland hormones effect the secretion of hypothalamic hormones in the same way that they effect the secretion of pituitary hormones, thereby reinforcing their effect on the production of the pituitary hormone.

The importance of the second negative feedback loop lies in the fact that the nerve cells of the hypothalamus receive impulses from other regions of the brain, including the cerebral cortex (the centre for higher mental functions, movement, perceptions, emotion, etc.), thus permitting the endocrine system to respond to physical and emotional stresses. This response mechanism involves the interruption of the primary feedback loop to allow the serum concentrations of hormones to be increased or decreased in response to environmental stresses that activate the nervous system (see below The hypothalamus). The end result of the two negative feedback loops is that, under ordinary circumstances, hormone production by target glands and the serum concentrations of target gland hormone are maintained within very narrow limits but that, under extraordinary circumstances, this tight control can be overridden by stimuli originating outside of the endocrine system.

There are important supplemental mechanisms that control endocrine function. When more than one cell type is found within a single endocrine gland, the hormones secreted by one cell type may exert a direct modulating effect upon the secretions of the other cell types. This form of control is known as paracrine control. Similarly, the secretions of one endocrine cell may alter the activity of the same cell, an activity known as autocrine control. Thus, endocrine cell activity may be modulated directly from within the endocrine gland itself, without the need for hormones to enter the bloodstream.

If the requirement that a hormone act at a site remote from the endocrine cells in which the hormone is produced is excluded from the defining characteristics of hormones, additional classes of biologically active materials can be considered as hormones. Neurotransmitters, a group of chemical compounds of variable composition, are secreted at all synapses (junctions between nerve cells over which nervous impulses must travel). They facilitate or inhibit the transmission of neural impulses and have given rise to the science of neuroendocrinology (the branch of medicine that studies the interaction of the nervous system and the endocrine system). A second group of biologically active substances is called prostaglandins. Prostaglandins are a complex group of fatty acid derivatives that are produced and secreted by many tissues. Prostaglandins mediate important biological effects in almost every organ system of the body.

Another group of substances, called growth factors, possess hormonelike activity. Growth factors are substances that stimulate the growth of specific tissues. They are distinct from pituitary growth hormone in that they were identified only after it was noted that target cells grown outside the organism in tissue culture could be stimulated to grow and reproduce by extracts of serum or tissue chemically distinct from growth hormone.

Still another area of hormonal activity that has come under intensive investigation is the effect of endocrine hormones on behaviour. While simple direct hormonal effects on human behaviour are difficult to document because of the complexities of human motivation, there are many convincing demonstrations of hormone-mediated behaviour in other life-forms. A special case is that of the pheromone, a substance generated by an organism that influences, by its odour, the behaviour of another organism of the same species. An often-quoted example is the musky scent of the females of many species, which provokes sexual excitation in the male. Such mechanisms have adaptive value for species survival.

Adrenal Glands

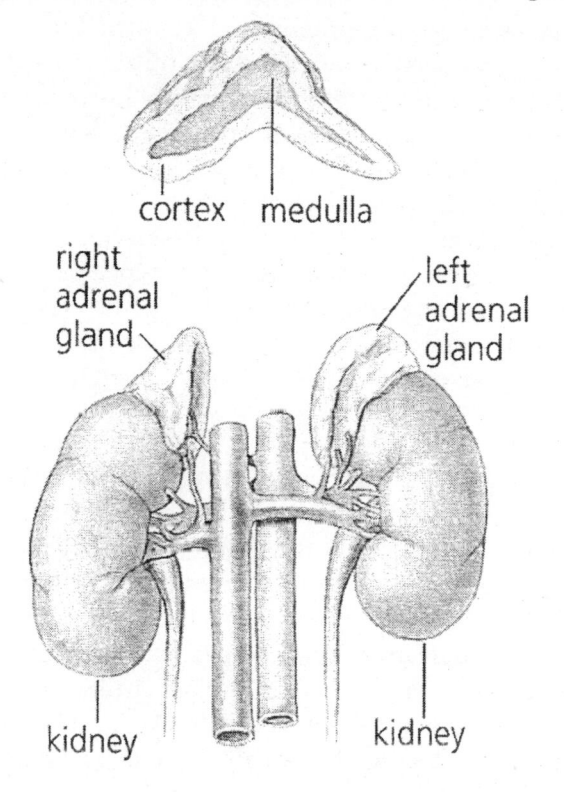

The adrenal glands are a pair of glands that secrete hormones directly into the bloodstream. Each gland can be divided into two distinct organs. The outer region secretes hormones which have important effects on the way in which energy is stored and food is used, on chemicals in the blood, and on characteristics such as hairiness and body shape. The smaller, inner region is part of the sympathetic nervous system and is the body's first line of defense and response to physical and emotional stresses. The adrenal glands are shaped like the French Emperor Napoleon's hat and, just as Napoleon's three-cornered hat sat on his head, so each gland is perched on each of the kidneys. These glands are about one to two inches in length and weigh only a fraction of an ounce each while secreting more than three dozen hormones. They take instruction from the pituitary glands and have important effects on physical characteristics, development and growth. The adrenal gland has two parts. The cortex, or outer, yellow layer, takes its instructions from the pituitary hormone ACTH. The hormones secreted here are called "steroids" and have three main types: those which control the balance of sodium and potassium in the body; those which raise the level of sugar in the blood; and sex hormones. The inner, reddish brown layer makes two types of hormones and takes all its instructions from the nervous system, producing chemicals which react to fear and anger and are sometimes called "fight or flight" hormones.

Ovaries

The ovaries are a pair of oval or almond-shaped glands which lie on either side of the uterus and just below the opening to the fallopian tubes. In addition to producing eggs or "ova," the ovaries produce female sex hormones called estrogen and progesterone. The ovaries produce a female hormone, called estrogen, and store female sex cells or "ova." The female, unlike the male, does not manufacture the sex cells. A girl baby is born with about 60,000 of these cells, which are contained

Fallopian tube
Ovary
Uterus
Cervix
Vagina

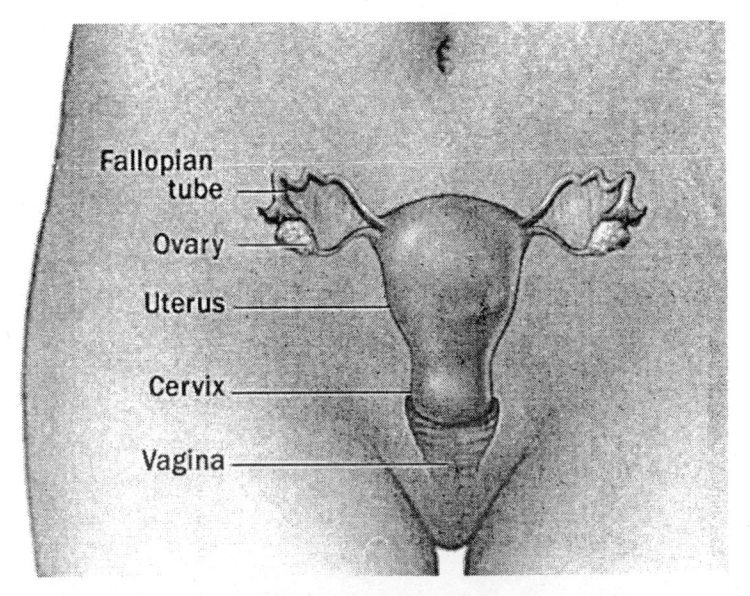

in sac-like depressions in the ovaries. Each of these cells may have the potential to mature for fertilization, but in actuality, only about 400 ripen during the woman's lifetime. Pregnant and prenatal both come from the same Latin roots. "Prae" means "before" and "nascor" means "to be born". Nascor is also the derivative of nature, innate and native. Only a few years ago, the word, "pregnant" was seldom used in mixed company. Polite society referred to a pregnant woman as "expecting" or "being in the family way."

Pancreas

The pancreas is a long. tapered gland which lies across and behind the stomach. The "head" (the right-hand end which is the broadest part of it) lies within the curve of the duodenum. This gland secretes digestive juices which break down fats, carbohydrates, proteins and acids; it also secretes bicarbonate, which neutralizes stomach acid as it enters the duodenum. Some cells in the pancreas secrete hormones which regulate the level

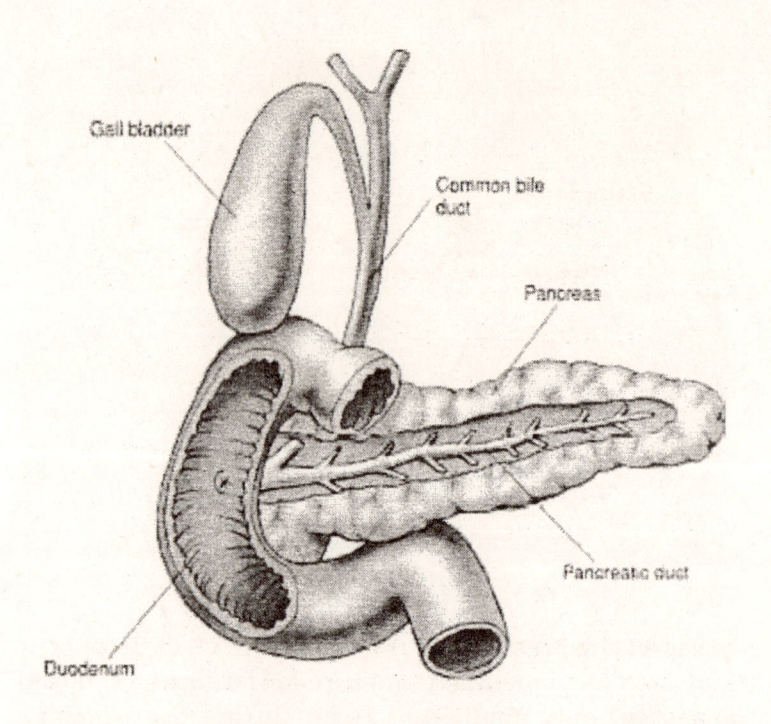

Figure: Gall bladder, Common bile duct, Pancreas, Pancreatic duct, Duodenum.

of glucose in the blood. Most of the pancreas consists of tissues which are embedded in "nested" cells. These cells secrete the digestive enzymes into tubes which meet to form the main duct. This duct joins the "cystic" duct (which carries bile from the gallbladder) and forms a small chamber which opens into the duodenum. The cells of the pancreas are surrounded by many blood vessels into which they secrete hormones (glucagon and insulin) into the blood. Insulin regulates the use of glucose into all the body tissues except the brain. If the pancreas fails to produce insulin or secretes it in low quantities, the result is a serious disease called diabetes mellitus. The Greek name "pancreas", meaning "all flesh" or "all meat", is descriptive of the protein composition of this powerful organ which resembles a fish with a large head and a long tail. Inside, the organ's appearance resembles a stalk with clusters of grapes attached to it.

The "stalk" is a long duct which runs down the center of the pancreas and the "grapes" are clusters of cells which flow into this duct and later into the duodenum for digestion of proteins, fats and carbohydrates. If the ducts leading from the pancreas are blocked in some way, the digestive fluids build up in the pancreas and may then become activated so that they digest the pancreas itself! This condition is known as acute pancreatitis. Pancreatic cancer has the worst prognosis of all the types of cancer. This is probably because of the spongy, vascular nature of this organ and its vital endocrine and exocrine functions. Pancreatic surgery is a problem because of the soft, spongy, tissue it consists of that make it extremely difficult to suture. By the way, Webster's Dictionary says the "pancratium" was an ancient Greek athletic contest involving boxing and wrestling. Isn't that interesting?

EXCRETORY SYSTEM

The excretory system is a biological system that removes excess, unnecessary or dangerous materials from an organism. It is responsible for the elimination of oxygen waste products of metabolism as well as other nitrogeneous materials. Since the normal operation of most biological systems creates waste, the excretory system is not necessarily distinct from other systems. Instead, it often represents the various excretory processes of several different systems.

Excretory Functions

Every organism, from the smallest protist to the largest mammal, must rid itself of the potentially harmful by-products of its own vital activities. This process in living things is called elimination, which may be considered to encompass all of the various mechanisms and processes by which life forms dispose of or throw off waste products, toxic substances, and dead portions of the organism. Egestion is the act of excreting unusable or undigested material from a cell (as opposed to metabolized waste), as in the case of single-celled organisms, or from the digestive tract of multi-cellular organisms.

As defined above, elimination broadly defines the mechanisms of waste disposal by living systems at all levels of complexity. The term may be used interchangeably with excretion, though not all elimination necessarily takes place in the excretory system.

Component Organs
Skin

The skin is another part of the excretory system: it eliminates sweat that helps cool the body and regulate the concentration of salt. The salt helps evaporate the water, cooling off the skin.

Liver

The liver is an organ of the digestive system. It also helps in excreting wastes from the body in a variety of processes. Laboratory analysis reveals a high concentration of a small organelle called a peroxisome, responsible for breakdown of several toxic substances. It also takes in nitrogenous wastes and converts them to urea to reduce their toxicity.

The liver absorbs drugs and other poisonous substances in the blood and changes their chemical structure to make them less toxic and easier to digest. This waste product is called bile and is excreted to the digestive tract, facilitating digestion of fats while also disposing of waste.

Kidneys

The key organs in the excretory system of vertebrates. The kidneys are placed on either side of the spinal column near the lower back. They are primarily responsible for filtering blood by removing nitrogenous wastes, though they also regulate blood pressure in a process called osmoregulation and also assist with the production of red blood cells.

Secretion

Secretion is the process of producing a substance from the cells and fluids within a gland or organ and discharging it.

The Ureters, Urinary Bladder, and Urethra

The two ureters conduct urine, by way of gravity and peristalsis, to the urinary bladder. The ureters enter the urinary bladder on the posterior surface at the top two corners of the trigone, a smooth, triangular shaped area of the urinary bladder floor. The urinary bladder is a hollow, muscular organ that functions in the temporary storage of urine. In males, the urinary bladder lies between the public symphysis and the rectum. In females, it is posterior to the public symphysis, inferior to the uterus, and superior to the vagina.

The inner wall contains folds called rugae that allow expansion and shrinkage of the bladder as it fills and empties with urine. A single duct, the urethra, drains urine from the bladder out of the body. Around the opening to the urethra are two sphincter muscles, the internal and external urethral sphincters. The internal urethral sphincter consists of smooth muscle and is therefore under involuntary nerve control. The external urethral sphincter is skeletal muscle tissue and under voluntary control.

This sphincter enables you to control the release of urine from the urinary bladder. As the bladder fills and expands with urine, stretch receptors signal motor neurons in the spinal cord to relax the internal urethral sphincter and contract the detrusor muscle of the bladder wall. This reflex automatically causes closing of the external urethral sphincter. When convenient, the external urethral sphincter is relaxed and urination, or micturition, occurs.

PHYSIOLOGY OF THE URINARY SYSTEM

The kidneys remove metabolic waste products such as toxin, excess water, and electrolytes from the blood plasma. Three physiological processes occur in the nephrons to maintain the composition of the blood and produce urine: filtration, reabsorption, and secretion. Filtration occurs in the renal corpuscle as blood pressure in the glomerulus forces water, small solutes, and ions out of the blood plasma and into the capsular space. The resulting fluid in the capsular space is called filtrate. Solute small enough to pass through the membranes of the renal corpuscle will appear in the filtrate. This results in a removal of both wastes and essential solutes from the blood.

The essential solutes and most of the water are returned to the blood by a process called reabsorption. Additionally, secretion by cells of the distal convoluted tubule occurs to add excess materials such as hydrogen and ammonium ions to the filtrate for excretion in the urine. As the filtrate passes through the tubules of the nephron, reabsorption and secretion occur. The modified filtrate, now called urine, drips out of the renal papillae into the minor calyxes. As the filtrate moves through the proximal convoluted tubule, 60% to 70% of the water, nutrients, and ions in the filtrate are reabsorbed into the blood. The cells of this tubule are simple cuboidal epithelium with microvilli to increase the lumen's surface area for reabsorption. The kidneys

Endocrine and Excretory System

filter 25% of the body's blood per minute, 24 hours a day. Approximately 180 litres of filtrate are formed by the glomerulus per day, which eventually results in the production of an average daily urinary output of between 1.0 and 2.0 litres of urine. The composition of urine can change daily depending on one's metabolic rate and urinary output. Water accounts for about 95% of the volume of urine. The other 5% contains excess water soluble vitamins, drugs, electrolytes, and nitrogenous wastes.

Urinalysis

Abnormal substances in urine can usually be detected by urinalysis, an analysis of the chemical and physical properties of urine. Test strips are a fast and inexpensive method of detecting the chemical composition of urine. Multistix and Chemstix are two popular brands of test strips. These sticks may contain from one to nine testing pads. Single test strips usually are used to detect if glucose or ketones are in the urine. The multiple test strips are used for a detailed analysis of the urine' chemical content. During this urinalysis, you will examine only your urine sample.

Physical characteristics such as volume, colour, cloudiness, and odour will be observed. The test strips will determine the chemical characteristics of your sample. Both physical and chemical properties of urine vary according to fluid intake and diet. Alternatively, you laboratory instructor may elect to provide your class with a mock urine sample for analysis. This artificial sample will probably include several abnormal constituents of urine for instructional purposes.

Composition of Urine

Normal constituents of urine include water; urea; creatinine; uric acid; many electrolytes; and possibly

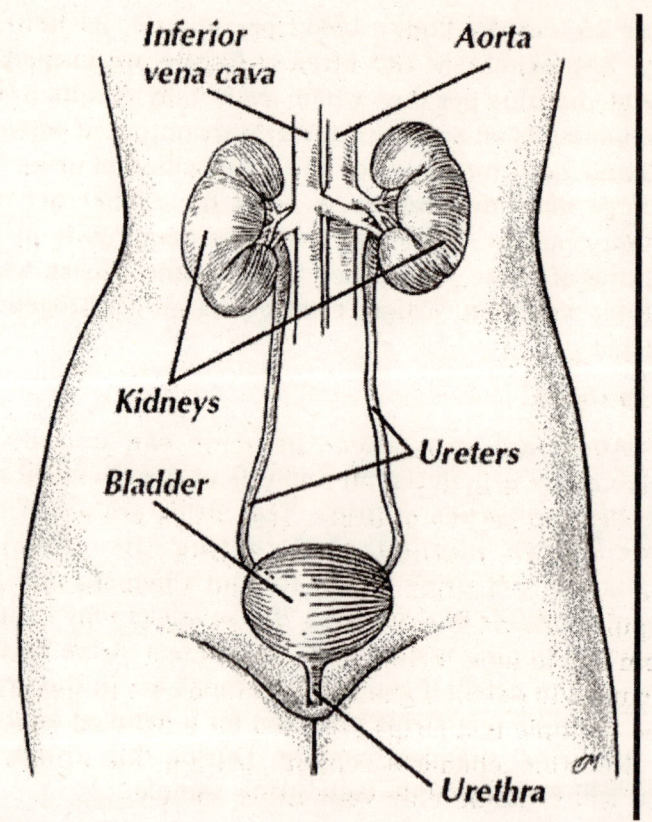

Inferior vena cava
Aorta
Kidneys
Ureters
Bladder
Urethra

small amounts of hormones, pigments, carbohydrates, fatty acids, mucin, and enzymes. Urea is produced during defemination reactions that remove ammonia from amino acids. The ammonia then combines with CO2 to form urea. About 1,800 milligrams of urea are produced daily. Urea makes up about 70% to 90% of all nitrogenous material in urine. Creatinine is formed from the breakdown of creatine phosphate, a molecule found associated with muscle tissue as an energy storage molecule. This material is entirely secreted and not reabsorbed. Uric acid is produced form the breakdown of the nucleic acids DNA and RNA from foods or cellular destruction. Several inorganic ions and molecules are also found in the urine.

Endocrine and Excretory System

Their presence is a reflection of diet and general health. Calcium, potassium, and magnesium ions are cations that form salts with chloride, sulfate, and phosphate ions. Na+ and Cl- are ions from sodium chloride, the principal salt of the body. Excretion of slat varies with their dietary intake. Ammonium is a product of protein catabolism and must be removed from the blood before it reaches toxic concentrations. Many types of ions bind with sodium and form a buffer in the blood and urine to stabilize fluid pH.

Other substances such as hormones, enzymes, carbohydrates, fatty acids, pigments, and mucin occur in small quantities in the urine. Abnormal materials in the urine suggest a disease process or an injury to the kidneys. Excessive consumption of certain substances causes a high concentration of that substance in the filtrate that saturates the transport mechanisms of reabsorption. Because the tubular cells cannot reclaim all the substance, it will appear in the urine.

Glucose

Glucose in the urine is usually an indication of diabetes mellitus. In this form of the disease, the individual produces an adequate amount of insulin. The body's cells, however, are less sensitive to the insulin because of a reduction in the number of insulin membrane receptors. As a result, excess levels of glucose are removed from the blood by the kidneys and voided in the urine.

Ketones

Ketones in the urine may be the result of starvation, diabetes mellitus, or a very low carbohydrate diet. When carbohydrate concentration in the blood is low, cells begin to catabolize fats. The products of fat catabolism are glycerol and fatty acids. Liver cells convert these fatty acids into ketone bodies that diffuse out of the liver cells and into the blood where they are filtered by the kidneys. In diabetes mellitus, commonly called sugar diabetes, sufficient amounts of glucose cannot enter cells. As a result, cells use fatty acids to produce ATP. This increase in fatty acid catabolism results in ketone bodies appearing in the urine.

Urobilinogen

Urobilinogen in the urine is called urobilinogenuria. Small amounts of urobilinogen in the urine are normal. It is a product of the breakdown of bilirubin by the intestines, and it is responsible for the normal brown colour of faces. Greater than trace levels in the urine may be due to infectious hepatitis, cirrhosis, congestive heart failure, or a variety or other diseases.

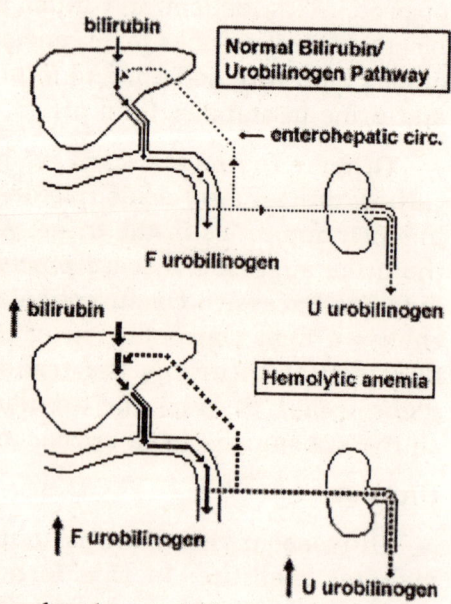

Albumin

Albumin is a large protein that normally cannot pass through filtering membranes of the glomerulus. A trace amount of albumin in the urine is urine is considered normal. Excessive albumin in the urine, a condition called albuminuria, suggests an increase in the permeability of the glomerular membrane. Reasons for the increased permeability could be the result of an injury, high blood pressure, disease, or the effect of bacterial toxins on the cells of the kidneys.

Microbes

Microbes in large numbers in the urine usually indicate an infection. Generally, urine is sterile, but microbe content is possible in a urine sample for several reasons. Microbes may contaminate a urine sample owing to their presence at the urethral opening and in the urethra.

Specific Gravity

Specific gravity of a fluid is a comparison of the density of that fluid to the density of water. The density of a fluid is the ratio of the weight of the solutes compared to the volume of the solvent. The specific gravity of water is 1.000. The average specific gravity for a normal urine sample is between 1.003 and 1.030, a density greater than water. Normal constituents of urine include water, urea, creatinine, sodium, chloride, potassium, sulphates, phosphates, and ammonium salts. These solutes determine the specific gravity of urine. High fluid intake results in frequent urination of a dilute urine with a lower specific gravity. Low fluid intake results in a more concentrated urine with a higher specific gravity. Excessively concentrated urine results in the crystallization of solutes into renal calculi or kidney stones.

Bilirubin

Bilirubin in large amounts in the urine, or bilirubinuria, is the result of the breakdown of haemoglobin from old red blood cells that are being removed from the circulatory system by phagocytic cells in the liver.

9

Digestive System

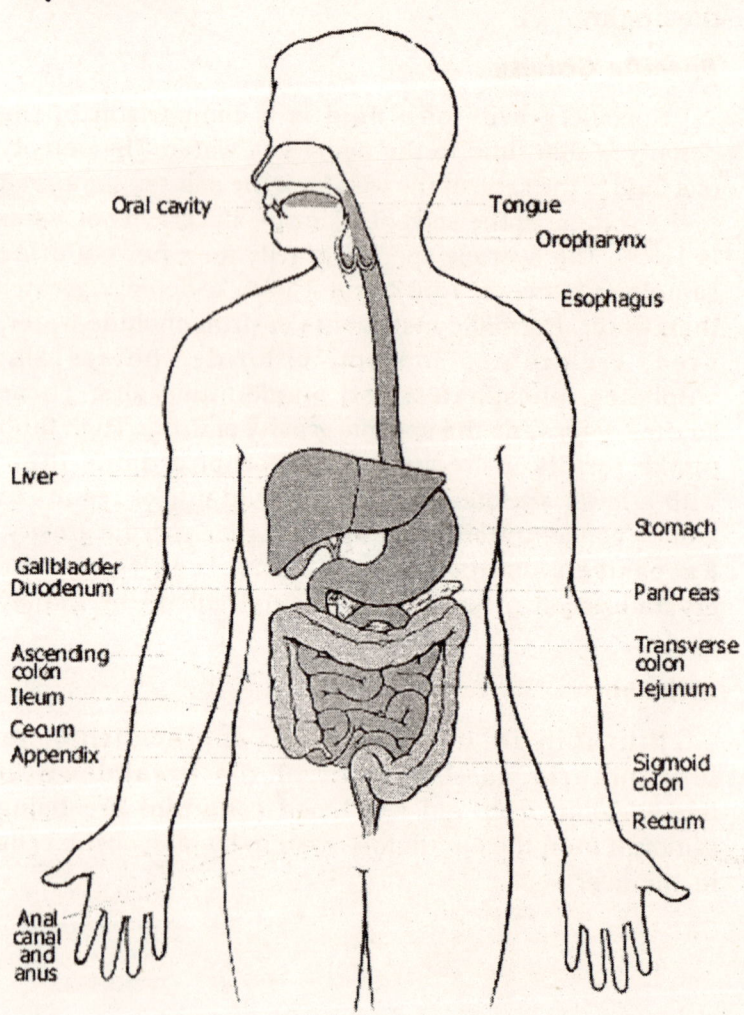

Digestive System

The digestive system processes food into usable forms for cellular metabolism. The digestive process includes (1) ingestion of food into the mouth, (2) movement of food through the digestive tract, (3) digestion of food by mechanical and enzymatic activities, (4) absorption of nutrients into the blood, and (5) formation and elimination of indigestible material and waste. To accomplish these functions, the digestive system is highly specialized. Food passes through a tubular digestive tract that extends from the mouth to the anus. Each organ of the tract has a specific function in the digestive process. Accessory organs, which include the salivary glands, liver, gallbladder, and pancreas, occur outside the digestive tract. These organs manufacture enzymes and other compounds that help in the digestive process. In this exercise, you will study the structure of the digestive organs. The digestive physiology section includes enzyme experiments to simulate the chemical breakdown of food.

Organization of the Digestive Tract

Examine the inside of your cheek with your tongue. What do you feel? The lining of your mouth and the rest of your digestive tract is a mucous membrane that is kept wet. Glands drench the lining epithelium with enzymes, mucus, pH buffers, and other compounds to orchestrate the sequential breakdown of food as it passes through your mouth, pharynx, oesophagus, stomach, small intestine, large intestine, and finally, rectum. Hormones secreted by the digestive tract regulate the digestive tract, the mucosa, submucosa, muscularis externa, and serosa. Although the basic histological structure of the tract is similar along its entire length, each region has anatomical specializations that reflect that region's role in the digestive process. The mucosa lines the lumen of the digestive tract and is in contact

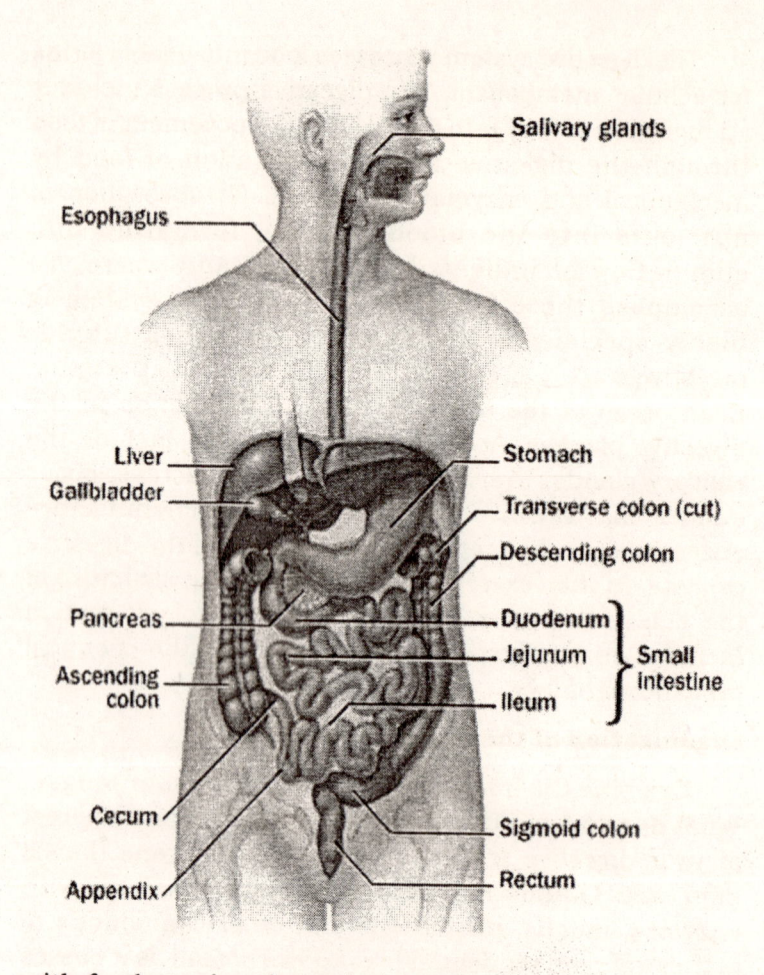

Diagram labels: Salivary glands, Esophagus, Liver, Gallbladder, Pancreas, Ascending colon, Cecum, Appendix, Stomach, Transverse colon (cut), Descending colon, Duodenum, Jejunum, Ileum, Small intestine, Sigmoid colon, Rectum

with food passing through the tract.

The mucosa consists of epithelial and connective tissues and a thin sheet of smooth muscle tissue. The mucosa is the only layer exposed to the lumen of the tract. From the mouth to the oesophagus, the epithelium is stratified squamous epithelium. Food passing from the mouth to the stomach is still in a solid condition, and the stratified epithelium protects the mucosa from abrasion. The stomach, small intestine, and large intestine are lined with simple columnar epithelium. Food in these parts of the tract is liquid and less abrasive to the digestive epithelium. Beneath the epithelium is a layer of connective tissue that attaches the epithelium and contains blood vessels, lymphatic vessels, and nerves. Superficial to the mucosa is the submucosa, a loose connective tissue layer containing large blood and lymphatic vessels and many nerves.

Surrounding the submucosa are several layers of smooth muscle tissue in the muscularis externa that move and process materials in the digestive tract. The inner layer is circular muscle that wraps outer layer is longitudinal muscle with fibres oriented parallel to the length of the tract. Contraction of this muscle layer shortens and widens the tract. Between the muscle layers are nerves that control the activity of the muscularis externa.

The Mouth

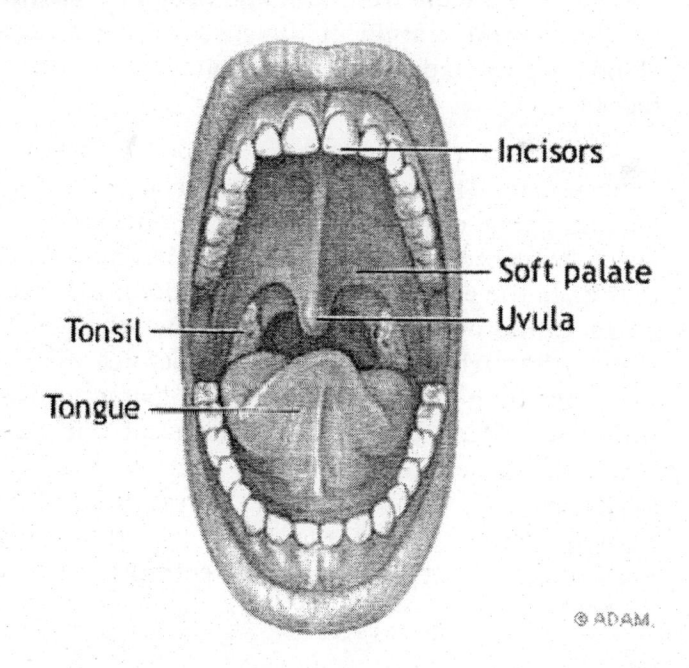

The mouth, or oral cavity, is the site of ingestion and the initial processing of food. The oral cavity extends from the labia to the faces, the opening between the mouth and the throat. The roof of the oral cavity consists of the hard and soft palates. A conical uvula is suspended from the posterior soft plate just anterior to the fauces. The floor of the mouth is muscular, mostly from muscles of the tongue, and the cheeks from the sides. A fold of tissue, the lingual frenulum, anchors the tongue yet allows free movement for food processing and speech. Accessory structures of the mouth include the salivary glands and the teeth.

The parotid gland is the large salivary gland in front of the ear between the skin and the masseter muscle. The parotid duct pierces through the buccinator muscle and enters the oral cavity near the upper near the upper second molar. The submandibular gland is located under the mandible. The submandibular duct passes through the lingual frenulum and opens at the swelling on the central margin of this tissue. The sublingual glands are located under the tongue at the floor of the mouth.

Many lesser sublingual ducts open along the base of the tongue. The teeth are used to mechanically process food into smaller pieces. The tooth is anchored into the avelar bone of the jaw by a strong periodontal ligament that lines the embedded part of the tooth, the root. The crown is the portion of the tooth above the gingiva, or gums. Although a tooth has many distinct layers, only the inner pulp cavity is filled with a living tissues, the pulp. Supplying the pulp tissue are blood vessels, lymphatic vessels, and nerves, all of which enter the pulp cavity through the root canal. Surrounding the pulp cavity is dentin, a hard, non-living solid that composes most of the structural mass of a tooth. At the root, the dentin is covered by cementum, which attaches to the periodontal ligament.

The exposed crown is covered with enamel, the hardest substance produced by living organisms. Humans have two sets of teeth during life. The first set are the deciduous, which are replaced starting around the age of six by the permanent dentition. The permanent dentition consists of 32 teeth. Each quadrant or jaw quarter has a central incisor, a lateral incisor, a bicuspid or canine, two premolars, and three molars. The last molar is also called the wisdom tooth. The bicuspids are pointed for learning actions. The premolars and molars have large flat surfaces for grinding food into small pieces.

The Pharynx and Oesophagus

The pharynx is a musculomembranous passage that leads from the nose and mouth to the esophagus. The passage of food from the pharynx into the esophagus is the second stage of swallowing. When food is being swallowed, the larynx is closed off from the pharynx to keep food from getting into the respiratory tract. The throat or pharynx is a common passageway for nutrients and air. The pharynx is divided into three anatomical regions, the nasopharynx, oropharynx, and larynx gopharynx. During swallowing, or dilatation, muscles of the soft palate contract and close the passageway to the nasopharynx to prevent food from entering the nasal cavity. The inferior portion of the oropharynx area branches into the larynx of the respiratory system and the oesophagus that leads to the stomach. To prevent food from entering the respiratory passageways, the larynx has a flap called the epiglottis, which closes the larynx during swallowing. The food tube or oesophagus connects the pharynx to the stomach. It is inferior to the pharynx and posterior to the trachea, or windpipe. The oesophagus is approximately 25 cm long. The oesophagus pierces through the diaphragm and connects with the stomach in the abdominal cavity.

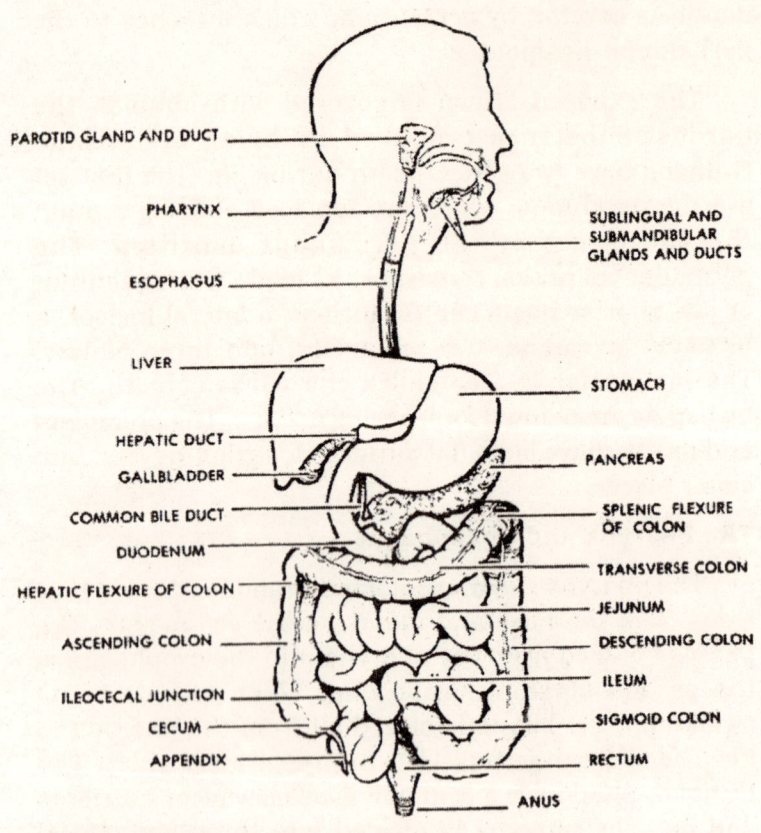

The Small Intestine and Large Intestine

The small intestine is approximately 21 feet long and consists of three segments: the duodenum, the jejunum, and the ileum. The first 10 inches, the duodenum, is attached to the distil region of the pylorus. The duodenum receives chyme from the stomach and digestive secretions from the liver, gallbladder, and pancreas. The jejunum is approximately 12 feet long and is the site of most nutrient absorption. The last region,

Digestive System

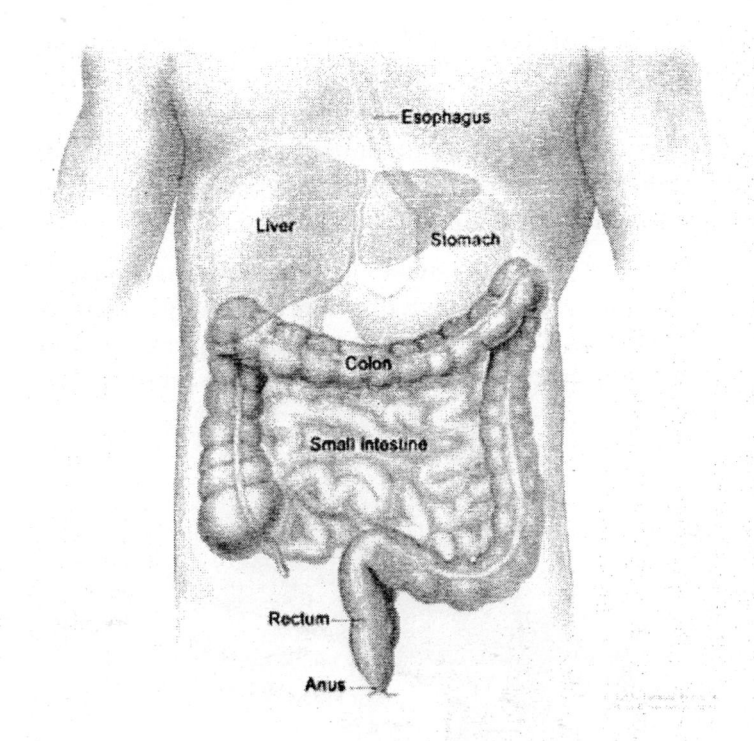

the ileum, ends at the leocecal valve, where it empties into the serum of the large intestine. The serosa or peritoneum of the small intestine of modified into sheets of tissue called mesentery, which support and attach the small intestine to the abdominal wall. The small intestine is the site of most digestive and absorptive activities and has specialized folds to increase surface area for these functions.

The submucosa and mucosa are creased together into large folds called plicae. Along the plicae, the mucosa is convoluted into finger like projections called villi. The large intestine is the site of water absorption and waste compaction. It is approximately 5 feet long and is divided into two groups, the colon and the rectum.

The first part of the colon, a puchlike serum, is located in the right iliac region. The ileocecal valve is at the junction of the ileum and serum. This sphincter muscle controls the movement of materials from the small intestine into several regions. The ascending colon travels up the right side of the abdomen.

It bends left to cross the abdomen below the stomach as the transverse colon, which then turns downward as the descending colon. The S-shaped sigmoid colon passes through the pelvic cavity to join the rectum. The

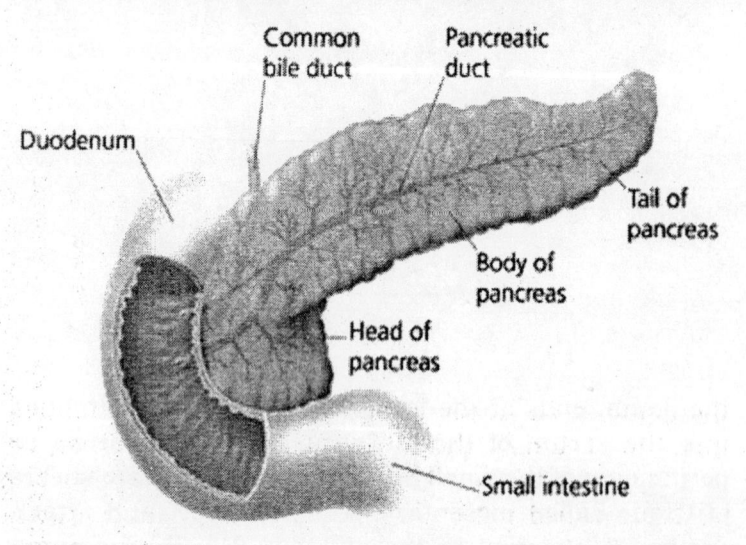

rectum, is the last 6 inches of the large intestine and the end of the digestive tract. The opening of the rectum is the anus, which is controlled by internal and external anal sphincters. The wall of the colon has many specializations. The longitudinal layer of the muscularis externa is reduced into three separate bands of muscle called the taenia coli. The tone of the taenia coli constrict the colon wall into paunches called haustrae. The haustrae allow expansion and stretching of the colon wall.

The Pancreas

The pancreas lies between the stomach and the duodenum. The pancreas is a "double" gland with endocrine and exocrine functions. The endocrine cells occur in pancreatic islets and secrete hormones for sugar metabolism. Most of the pancreatic cells consist of exocrine glands. Acinar cells secrete pancreatic juice rich in enzymes and buffers into the pancreatic duct that meets the common bile duct in the duodenal ampulla.

The Stomach

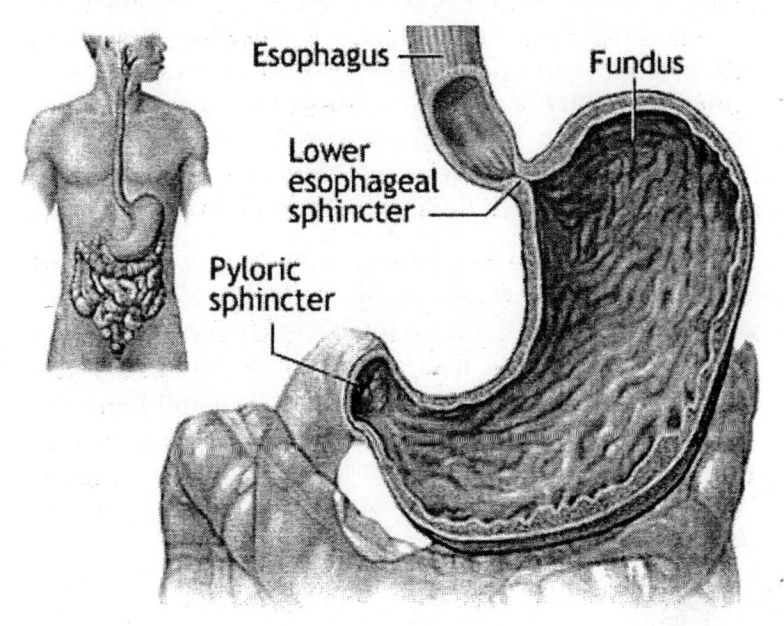

The stomach is a J-shaped organ located inferior to the diaphragm in the epigastric and lower left hypochondriac regions. The cardia is where the stomach connects with the oesophagus, the fundus is the upper rounded area, the body is the middle region, and the pylorus is the narrowed distil end that connects to the small intestine. The pyloric sphincter or valve controls movement of material from the stomach into the small intestine. Extending from the stomach is the greater omentum, a part of the serosa commonly called the fatty apron. This fatty layer protects the abdominal organs and attaches the transverse colon of the large intestine to the abdominal wall.

The lesser omentum suspends the stomach from the liver. The inner lining of the stomach has rugae or folds that enable the stomach to expand as it fills with food. Unlike other regions of the digestive tract, the muscularis external of the stomach contains three layers of smooth muscle instead of two. The inner layer is an oblique layer, followed by a circular layer, then an external longitudinal layer. The three muscle layers contract and churn the stomach contents into a soupy mixture called chyme.

The Liver and Gallbladder

The liver is located mostly in the right hypochondriac region, inferior to the diaphragm. Each lobe is divided into thousands of smaller lobulus, which we discuss in an upcoming section. The liver has a wide range of functions. It manufactures bile, a salt involved in fat digestion. Bile flows into right and left hepatic ducts, which merge to from a common hepatic duct. The gallbladder is located inferior to the right lobe of the liver.

It is a small muscular sac that stores and concentrates bile salts used is digestion of lipids. The common hepatic duct from the liver meets of cystic duct of the gallbladder to from the common bile duct. This duct passes through the lesser omentum and joins the pancreatic duct of the pancreas. These ducts enter the duodenum of the small intestine. A sphincter muscle regulates the flow of pancreatic juice and bile into the duodenum.

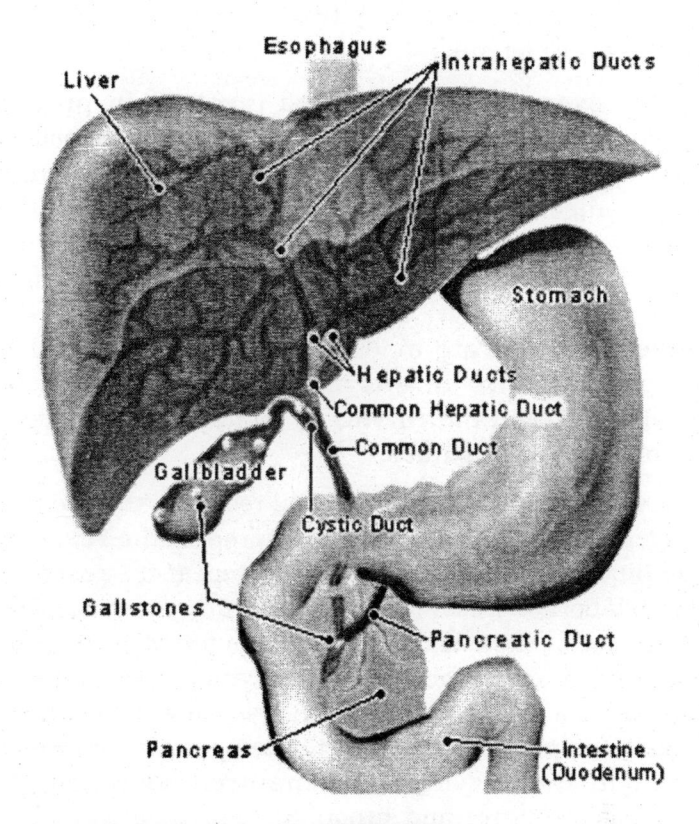

THE PHYSIOLOGY OF DIGESTION

Before nutrients can be converted into usable energy by cells, the large organic macro-molecules in food must be catabolized or broken down into monomers, the building blocks of macromolecules. These chemical reactions are controlled by enzymes produced by the digestive system. Enzymes are protein catalysts that lower activation energy, the energy required for a chemical reaction. Without enzymes, the body would have to heat up to dangerous temperatures to provide the activation energy necessary to decompose ingested food. Enzymes have a narrow range of physical conditions in which they operate at maximum efficiency.

Temperature and pH are two important factors of enzymatic reactions.

For example, the enzymes involved in protein digestion require a different pH. The enzyme pepsin is most active in acidic conditions of the stomach. The next protein-digesting enzyme in the sequence, trypsin, requires an alkaline environment. An enzymatic reaction involves reactants, called the substrate, and results in a product. The enzyme has an active site where the substrate binds. Only a substrate that is compatible with an enzyme's active site will be metabolized, and the enzyme is said to have specificity for compatible substrates.

On completion of the chemical reaction, the product is released and the enzyme, unaltered in the reaction, may bind to another substrate and repeat the reaction. In this laboratory exercise, you will study the conditions necessary for the enzymatic reactions for carbohydrate, lipid, and protein digestion. All enzyme experiments in this exercise will be incubated in a warm water bath set at body temperature, 37°C. If the temperature becomes too high, the enzyme will denature, destroying its chemical structure and function.

10

Sensory System

A sensory system is a part of the nervous system responsible for processing sensory information. A sensory system consists of sensory receptors, neural pathways, and parts of the brain involved in sensory perception. Commonly recognized sensory systems are those for vision, hearing, somatic sensation (touch), taste and olfaction (smell).

The receptive field is the specific part of the world to which a receptor organ and receptor cells respond. For instance, the part of the world an eye can see, is its receptive field; the light that each rod or cone can see, is its receptive field. Receptive fields have been identified for the visual system, auditory system and somatosensory system, so far.

Stimulus

Sensory systems code for four aspects of a stimulus; type (modality), intensity, location, and duration. Arrival time of a sound pulse and phase differences of continuous sound are used for localization of sound sources. Certain receptors are sensitive to certain types of stimuli (for example, different mechanoreceptors respond best to different kinds of touch stimuli, like sharp or blunt objects). Receptors send impulses in certain patterns to send information about the intensity of a stimulus (for example, how loud a sound is). The location of the receptor that is stimulated gives the brain information about the location of the stimulus (for example, stimulating a mechanoreceptor in a finger will send information to the brain about that finger). The duration of the stimulus (how long it lasts) is conveyed by firing patterns of receptors.

Modality

A stimulus modality (sensory modality) is a type of physical phenomenon that can be sensed. Examples are temperature, taste, sound, and pressure. The type of sensory receptor activated by a stimulus plays the primary role in coding the stimulus modality.

In the memory-prediction framework, Jeff Hawkins mentions a correspondence between the six layers of the cerebral cortex and the six layers of the optic tract of the visual system. The primary visual cortex has areas labelled V1, V2, V3, V4, V5, MT, IT, etc. Thus Area V1 mentioned below, is meant to signify only one class of cells in the brain, for which there can be many other cells which are also engaged in vision.

Hawkins lays out a scheme for the analogous modalities of the sensory system. Note that there can be many types of senses, some not mentioned here. In particular, for humans, there will be cells which can be labelled as belonging to V1, V2 A1, A2, etc.:

V1 (Vision)

Visual Area 1, or V1, is used for vision, via the visual system to the primary visual cortex.

A1 (Auditory - Hearing)

Auditory Area 1, or A1, is for hearing, via the auditory system, the primary auditory cortex.

S1 (Somatosensory - Touch)

Somatosensory Area 1, or S1, is for touch and

proprioception in the somatosensory system. The somatosensory system feeds the Brodmann Areas 3, 1 and 2 of the primary somatosensory cortex. But there are also pathways for proprioception (via the cerebellum), and motor control (via Brodmann area 4).

Tongue

G1 (gustatory - taste)

Gustatory Area 1, or G1, is used for taste.

O1 (olfactory - smell)

Olfactory Area 1, or O1, is used for smell. In contrast to vision and hearing, the olfactory bulbs are not cross-hemispheric; the right bulb connects to the right hemisphere and the left bulb connects to the left hemisphere.

VISUAL SYSTEM

The visual system is the part of the central nervous system which enables organisms to see. It interprets the information from visible light to build a representation of the world surrounding the body. The visual system

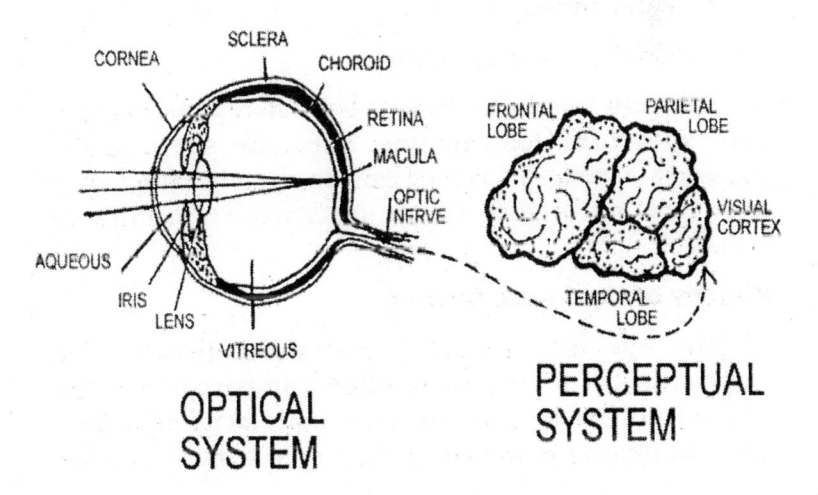

OPTICAL SYSTEM

PERCEPTUAL SYSTEM

accomplishes a number of complex tasks, including the reception of light, and the formation of monocular representations; the construction of a binocular perception from a pair of two dimensional projections; the identification and categorization of visual objects; assessing distances to and between objects; and guiding body movements to visual objects. The psychological manifestation of visual information is known as visual perception.

The present study mostly describes the visual system of mammals, although other "higher" animals have similar visual systems. In this case, the visual system consists of:

- The eye, especially the retina
- The optic nerve
- The optic chiasma
- The optic tract
- The lateral geniculate body
- The optic radiation
- Visual cortex
- Visual association cortex

Different species are able to see different parts of the light spectrum; for example, bees can see into the ultraviolet, while pit vipers can accurately target prey with their pit organs, which are sensitive to infrared radiation.

Biology of the Visual System

The eye is a complex biological device. The functioning of a camera is often compared with the workings of the eye, mostly since both focus light from external objects in the visual field onto a light-sensitive medium. In the case of the camera, this medium is film or an electronic sensor; in the case of the eye, it is an array of visual receptors. With this simple geometrical similarity, based on the laws of optics, the eye functions as a transducer, as does a CCD camera.

Light entering the eye is refracted as it passes through the cornea. It then passes through the pupil (controlled by the iris) and is further refracted by the lens. The cornea and lens act together as a compound lens to project an inverted image onto the retina.

Retina

The retina consists of a large number of photoreceptor cells which contain a particular protein molecule called an opsin. In humans, two types of opsins are involved in vision: rod opsins and cone opsins. (A third type, melanopsin in some of the retinal ganglion cells, part of the body clock mechanism, is probably not involved in vision.) An opsin absorbs a photon (a particle of light) and transmits a signal to the cell through a signal transduction pathway, resulting in hyperpolarization of the photoreceptor.

Rods and cones differ in function. Rods are found primarily in the periphery of the retina and are used to see at low levels of light. Cones are found primarily in the center (or fovea) of the retina. There are three types of cones that differ in the wavelengths of light they absorb; they are usually called short or blue, middle or green, and long or red. Cones are used primarily to distinguish color and other features of the visual world at normal levels of light.

In the retina, the photoreceptors synapse directly onto bipolar cells, which in turn synapse onto ganglion cells of the outermost layer, which will then conduct action potentials to the brain. A significant amount of visual processing arises from the patterns of communication between neurons in the retina. About 130 million photoreceptors absorb light, yet roughly 1.2 million axons of ganglion cells transmit information from the retina to the brain. The processing in the retina includes the formation of center-surround receptive fields of bipolar and ganglion cells in the retina, as well as convergence and divergence from photoreceptor to bipolar cell. In addition, other neurons in the retina, particularly horizontal and amacrine cells, transmit information laterally (from a neuron in one layer to an adjacent neuron in the same layer), resulting in more complex receptive fields that can be either indifferent to color and sensitive to motion or sensitive to color and indifferent to motion.

The final result of all this processing is five different populations of ganglion cells that send visual (image-forming and non-image-forming) information to the brain:

1. M cells, with large center-surround receptive fields that are sensitive to depth, indifferent to color, and rapidly adapt to a stimulus;

2. P cells, with smaller center-surround receptive fields that are sensitive to color and shape;

3. K cells, with very large center-only receptive fields that are sensitive to color and indifferent to shape or depth;

4. another population that is intrinsically photosensitive; and

5. a final population that is used for eye movements.

A 2006 University of Pennsylvania study calculated the approximate bandwidth of human retinas to be about 8960 kilobits per second, whereas guinea pig retinas transfer at about 875 kilobits.

In 2007 Zaidi and co-researchers on both sides of the Atlantic studying patients without rods and cones, discovered that the novel photoreceptive ganglion cell in humans also has a role in conscious and unconscious visual perception. The peak spectral sensitivity was 481nm. This shows that there are two pathways for sight in the retina - one based on classic photoreceptors (rods and cones) and the other, newly discovered, based on photoreceptive ganglion cells which act as rudimentary visual brightness detectors.

Photochemistry

Visual Cycle

In the visual system, retinal, technically called retinene1 or "retinaldehyde", is a light-sensitive retinene molecule found in the rods and cones of the retina. Retinal is the fundamental structure involved in the transduction of light into visual signals, i.e. nerve impulses in the ocular system of the central nervous system. In the presence of light, the retinal molecule changes configuration and as a result a nerve impulse is generated.

Fibres to Thalamus

Optic Nerve

Information flow from the eyes (top), crossing at the optic chiasma, joining left and right eye information in the optic tract, and layering left and right visual stimuli in the lateral geniculate nucleus. V1 in red at bottom of image. The information about the image via the eye is transmitted to the brain along the optic nerve. Different populations of ganglion cells in the retina send information to the brain through the optic nerve. About 90% of the axons in the optic nerve go to the lateral geniculate nucleus in the thalamus. These axons originate from the M, P, and K ganglion cells in the retina, see above. This parallel processing is important for reconstructing the visual world; each type of information will go through a different route to perception. Another population sends information to the superior colliculus in the midbrain, which assists in controlling eye movements (saccades).

A final population of photosensitive ganglion cells, containing melanopsin, sends information via the retinohypothalamic tract (RHT) to the pretectum (pupillary reflex), to several structures involved in the control of circadian rhythms and sleep such as the suprachiasmatic nucleus (SCN, the biological clock), and to the ventrolateral preoptic nucleus (VLPO, a region involved in sleep regulation). A recently discovered role for photoreceptive ganglion cells is that they mediate conscious and unconscious vision - acting as rudimentary visual brightness detectors shown in rodless coneless eyes.

Optic Chiasm

The optic nerves from both eyes meet and cross at the optic chiasm, at the base of the hypothalamus of the brain. At this point the information coming from both eyes is combined and then splits according to the visual field. The corresponding halves of the field of view (right and left) are sent to the left and right halves of the brain, respectively, to be processed. That is, the right side of primary visual cortex deals with the left half of the field of view from both eyes, and similarly for the left brain. A small region in the center of the field of view is processed redundantly by both halves of the brain.

Optic Tract

Information from the right visual field (now on the

left side of the brain) travels in the left optic tract. Information from the left visual field travels in the right optic tract. Each optic tract terminates in the lateral geniculate nucleus (LGN) in the thalamus.

Six layers in the LGN

Lateral Geniculate Nucleus

The lateral geniculate nucleus (LGN) is a sensory relay nucleus in the thalamus of the brain. The LGN consists of six layers in humans and other primates starting from catarhinians, including cercopithecidae and apes. Layers 1, 4, and 6 correspond to information from the contralateral (crossed) fibers of the nasal visual field; layers 2, 3, and 5 correspond to information from the ipsilateral (uncrossed) fibers of the temporal visual field. Layer one (1) contains M cells, which correspond to the M (magnocellular) cells of the optic nerve of the opposite eye, and are concerned with depth or motion. Layers four and six (4 & 6) of the LGN also connect to the opposite eye, but to the P cells (color and edges) of the optic nerve. By contrast, layers two, three and five (2, 3, & 5) of the LGN connect to the M cells and P (parvocellular) cells of the optic nerve for the same side of the brain as its respective LGN. The six layers of the LGN are the area of a credit card, but about three times the thickness of a credit card, rolled up into two ellipsoids about the size and shape of two small birds eggs. In between the six layers are smaller cells that receive information from the K cells (color) in the retina. The neurons of the LGN then relay the visual image to the primary visual cortex (V1) which is located at the back of the brain (caudal end) in the occipital lobe in and close to the calcarine sulcus.

Gray's FIG. 722– Scheme showing central connections of the optic nerves and optic tracts.

Optic Radiation

The optic radiations carries information from the thalamic lateral geniculate nucleus to layer 4 of the visual cortex. The P layer neurons of the LGN relay to V1 layer 4C ß. The M layer neurons relay to V1 layer 4C a. The K layer neurons in the LGN relay to large neurons called blobs in layers 2 and 3 of V1.

There is a direct correspondence from an angular position in the field of view of the eye, all the way through the optic tract to a nerve position in V1. At this juncture in V1, the image path ceases to be straightforward; there is more cross-connection within the visual cortex.

Visual Cortex

Visual cortex: V1, V2, V3, V4, V5 (also called MT)The visual cortex is the most massive system in the human brain and is responsible for processing the visual image. It lies at the rear of the brain (highlighted in the image), above the cerebellum. The region that receives information directly from the LGN is called the primary visual cortex, (also V1 and striate cortex). Visual information then flows through a cortical hierarchy. These areas include V2, V3, V4 and area V5/MT (the exact connectivity depends on the species of the animal). These secondary visual areas (collectively termed the extrastriate visual cortex) process a wide variety of visual primitives. Neurons in V1 and V2 respond selectively to bars of specific orientations, or combinations of bars. These are believed to support edge and corner detection. Similarly, basic information about color, motion is processed here.

Visual Association Cortex

Dorsal Stream

Ventral Stream

As visual information passes forward through the visual hierarchy, the complexity of the neural representations increase. Whereas a V1 neuron may respond selectively to a line segment of a particular orientation in a particular retinotopic location, neurons in the lateral occipital complex respond selectively to complete object (e.g., a figure drawing), and neurons in visual association cortex may respond selectively to human faces, or to a particular object. Along with this increased complexity comes specialization of two distinct pathways: the dorsal stream and the ventral stream. The dorsal stream, commonly referred to as the "where" stream, is involved in spatial attention, and communicates with regions that control eye movements and hand movements. More recently, this area has been called the "how" stream to emphasize its role in guiding behaviors to spatial locations. The ventral stream, commonly referred as the "what" stream, is involved in the recognition, identification and categorization of visual stimuli.

AUDITORY SYSTEM

The auditory system is the sensory system for the sense of hearing.

EAR

Anatomy of the human ear. (The length of the auditory canal is exaggerated in this image)

Outer Ear

The folds of cartilage surrounding the ear canal are called the pinna. Sound waves are reflected and attenuated when they hit the pinna, and these changes provide additional information that will help the brain determine the direction from which the sounds came.

The sound waves enter the auditory canal, a deceptively simple tube. The ear canal amplifies sounds

Basic Anatomy and Physiology

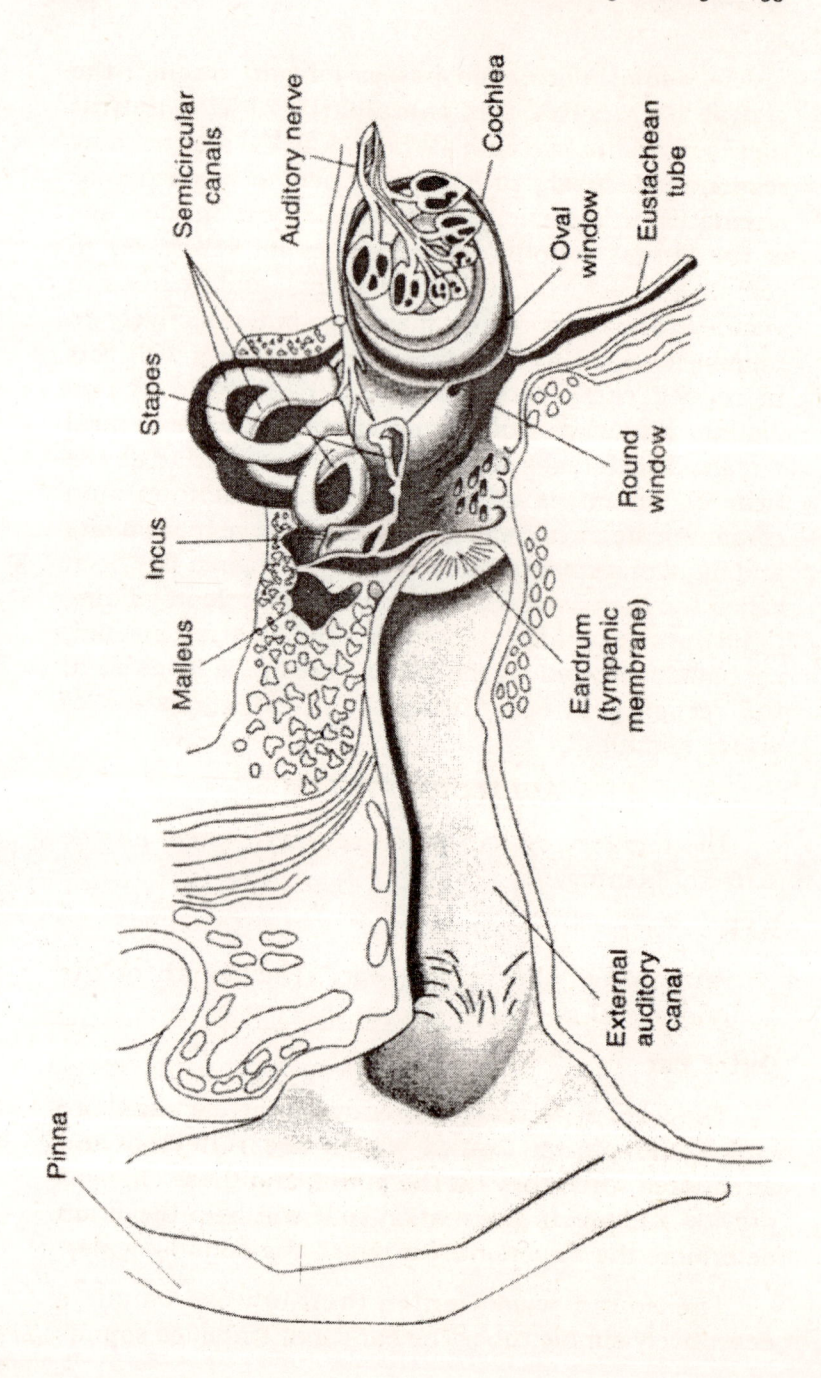

that are between 3 and 12 kHz. At the far end of the ear canal is the eardrum (or tympanic membrane), which marks the beginning of the middle ear.

Middle Ear

Sound waves traveling through the ear canal will hit the tympanic membrane, or eardrum. This wave information travels across the air-filled middle ear cavity via a series of delicate bones: the malleus (hammer), incus (anvil) and stapes (stirrup). These ossicles act as a lever and a teletype, converting the lower-pressure eardrum sound vibrations into higher-pressure sound vibrations at another, smaller membrane called the oval (or elliptical) window. The malleus articulates with the tympanic membrane via the manubrium, where the stapes articulates with the oval window via its footplate. Higher pressure is necessary because the inner ear beyond the oval window contains liquid rather than air. The sound is not amplified uniformly across the ossicular chain. The stapedius muscle reflex of the middle ear muscles helps protect the inner ear from damage. The middle ear still contains the sound information in wave form; it is converted to nerve impulses in the cochlea.

Inner Ear

Cochlea

Diagrammatic longitudinal section of the cochlea. Scala media is labeled as ductus cochlearis at right.

The inner ear consists of the cochlea and several non-auditory structures. The cochlea has three fluid-filled sections, and supports a fluid wave driven by pressure across the basilar membrane separating two of the sections. Strikingly, one section, called the cochlear duct or scala media, contains an extracellular fluid similar in composition to endolymph, which is usually found inside of cells. The organ of Corti is located at this duct, and transforms mechanical waves to electric signals in neurons. The other two sections are known as the scala tympani and the scala vestibuli, these are located within the bony labyrinth which is filled with fluid called perilymph. The chemical difference between the two fluids (endolymph & perilymph) is important for the function of the inner ear.

Organ of Corti

The organ of Corti forms a ribbon of sensory epithelium which runs lengthwise down the entire cochlea. The hair cells of the organ of Corti transform the fluid waves into nerve signals. The journey of a billion nerves begins with this first step; from here further processing leads to a panoply of auditory reactions and sensations.

The organ of Corti located at the scala media.

Hair Cell

Hair cells are columnar cells, each with a bundle of 100-200 specialized cilia at the top, for which they are named. These cilia are the mechanosensors for hearing. Lightly resting atop the longest cilia is the tectorial membrane, which moves back and forth with each cycle of sound, tilting the cilia and allowing electric current into the hair cell.

Hair cells, like the photoreceptors of the eye, show a graded response, instead of the spikes typical of other neurons. These graded potentials are not bound by the "all or none" properties of an action potential.

At this point, one may ask how such a wiggle of a hair bundle triggers a difference in membrane potential. The current model is that cilia are attached to one another by "tip links", structures which link the tips of one cilium to another. Stretching and compressing the tip links may open an ion channel and produce the receptor potential in the hair cell. Recently it has been shown that cdh23 and pchh15 are the adhesion molecules associated with these tip links. It is thought that a calcium driven motor causes a shortening of these links to regenerate tensions. This regeneration of tension allows for apprehension of prolonged auditory stimulation.

Neurons

Hair cell neural connection

Afferent neurons innervate cochlear inner hair cells, at synapses where the neurotransmitter glutamate communicates signals from the hair cells to the dendrites of the primary auditory neurons.

There are far fewer inner hair cells in the cochlea than afferent nerve fibers. The neural dendrites belong to neurons of the auditory nerve, which in turn joins the vestibular nerve to form the vestibulocochlear nerve, or cranial nerve number VIII.

Efferent projections from the brain to the cochlea also play a role in the perception of sound. Efferent synapses occur on outer hair cells and on afferent (towards the brain) dendrites under inner hair cells.

CENTRAL AUDITORY SYSTEM

This sound information, now re-encoded, travels down the vestibulocochlear nerve, through intermediate stations such as the cochlear nuclei and superior olivary complex of the brainstem and the inferior colliculus of the midbrain, being further processed at each waypoint. The information eventually reaches the thalamus, and from there it is relayed to the cortex. In the human brain, the primary auditory cortex is located in the temporal lobe.

Associated anatomical structures include:

Cochlear Nucleus

The cochlear nucleus is the first site of the neuronal processing of the newly converted "digital" data from the inner ear. This region is anatomically and physiologically split into two regions, the dorsal cochlear nucleus (DCN), and ventral cochlear nucleus (VCN).

Trapezoid Body

The Trapezoid body is a bundle of decussating fibers in the ventral pons that carry information used for binaural computations in the brainstem.

Superior Olivary Complex

The superior olivary complex is located in the pons, and receives projections predominantly from the ventral cochlear nucleus, although the posterior cochlear nucleus projects there as well, via the ventral acoustic stria. Within the superior olivary complex lies the lateral superior olive (LSO) and the medial superior olive (MSO). The former is important in detecting interaural level differences while the latter is important in distinguishing interaural time difference.

Lateral lemniscus in red, as it connects the cochlear nucleus, superior olivary nucleus and the inferior colliculus. Seen from behind.

Lateral Lemniscus

The lateral lemniscus is a tract of axons in the brainstem that carries information about sound from the cochlear nucleus to various brainstem nuclei and ultimately the contralateral inferior colliculus of the midbrain.

Inferior Colliculi

The IC are located just below the visual processing

centers known as the superior colliculi. The central nucleus of the IC is a nearly obligatory relay in the ascending auditory system, and most likely acts to integrate information (specifically regarding sound source localization from the superior olivary complex and dorsal cochlear nucleus) before sending it to the thalamus and cortex.

Medial Geniculate Nucleus

The medial geniculate nucleus is part of the thalamic relay system.

Primary Auditory Cortex

The primary auditory cortex is the first region of cerebral cortex to receive auditory input.

Perception of sound is associated with the right posterior superior temporal gyrus (STG). The superior temporal gyrus contains several important structures of the brain, including Brodmann areas 41 and 42, marking the location of the primary auditory cortex, the cortical region responsible for the sensation of basic characteristics of sound such as pitch and rhythm.

TASTE

"Sour" redirects here. For other uses, see Sour (disambiguation).

This article is about the sense. For the social and aesthetic aspects of "taste", see Taste (sociology). For other uses, see Taste (disambiguation).

Taste budTaste (or, more formally, gustation) is a form of direct chemoreception and is one of the traditional five senses. It refers to the ability to detect the flavor of substances such as food, certain minerals, and poisons. In humans and many other vertebrate animals the sense of taste partners with the less direct sense of smell, in the brain's perception of flavor. In the West, experts traditionally identified four taste sensations: sweet, salty, sour, and bitter. Eastern experts traditionally identified a fifth, called umami (savory). More recently, psychophysicists and neuroscientists have suggested other taste categories (umami and fatty acid taste most prominently, as well as the sensation of metallic and water tastes, although the latter is commonly disregarded due to the phenomenon of taste adaptation. Taste is a sensory function of the central nervous system. The receptor cells for taste in humans are found on the surface of the tongue, along the soft palate, and in the epithelium of the pharynx and epiglottis.

Overview

Psychophysicists have long suggested the existence of four taste 'primaries', referred to as the basic tastes: sweetness, bitterness, sourness and saltiness. Although first described in 1908, umami has been only recently recognized as the fifth basic taste since the cloning of a specific amino acid taste receptor in 2002. Umami taste is exemplified by the non-salty sensations evoked by some free amino acids such as monosodium glutamate.

Other possible categories have been suggested, such as a taste exemplified by certain fatty acids such as linoleic acid. Some researchers still argue against the notion of primaries at all and instead favor a continuum of percepts, similar to color vision.

All of these taste sensations arise from all regions of the oral cavity, despite the common misconception of a "taste map" of sensitivity to different tastes thought to correspond to specific areas of the tongue. This myth is generally attributed to the mistranslation of a German text, and perpetuated in North American schools since the early twentieth century. Very slight regional differences in sensitivity to compounds exist, though these regional differences are subtle and do not conform exactly to the mythical tongue map. Individual taste buds (which contain approximately 100 taste receptor cells), in fact, typically respond to compounds evoking each of the five basic tastes.

BASIC TASTES

For a long period, it has been commonly accepted that there are a finite number of "basic tastes" by which all foods and tastes can be grouped. Just like with primary colors, these "basic tastes" only apply to the human perception, ie. the different sorts of tastes our tongue can identify. Up until the 2000s, this was considered to be a group of four basic tastes. More recently, a fifth taste, Umami, has been proposed by a large number of authorities associated with this field.

Bitterness

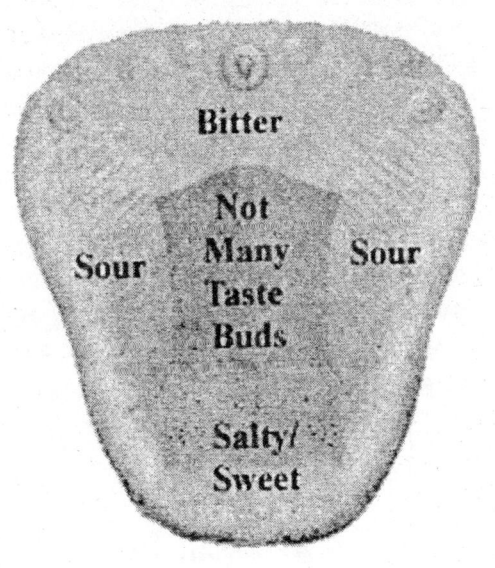

Bitterness is the most sensitive of the tastes, and is perceived by many to be unpleasant, sharp, or disagreeable. Common bitter foods and beverages include coffee, unsweetened chocolate, bitter melon, beer, bitters, olives, citrus peel, many plants in the Brassicaceae family, dandelion greens and escarole. Quinine is also known for its bitter taste and is found in tonic water.

Research has shown that TAS2Rs (taste receptors, type 2, also known as T2Rs) such as TAS2R38 coupled to the G protein gustducin are responsible for the human ability to taste bitter substances. They are identified not only by their ability to taste for certain "bitter" ligands, but also by the morphology of the receptor itself (surface bound, monomeric). Researchers use two synthetic substances, phenylthiocarbamide (PTC) and 6-n-propylthiouracil (PROP) to study the genetics of bitter perception. These two substances taste bitter to some people, but are virtually tasteless to others. Among the tasters, some are so-called "supertasters" to whom PTC and PROP are extremely bitter. This genetic variation in the ability to taste a substance has been a source of great interest to those who study genetics.

In addition, it is of interest to those who study evolution, as well as various health researchers since PTC-tasting is associated with the ability to taste numerous natural bitter compounds, a large number of which are known to be toxic. The ability to detect bitter-tasting, toxic compounds at low thresholds is considered to provide an important protective function. Plant leaves often contain toxic compounds, yet even amongst leaf-eating primates,there is a tendency to prefer immature leaves, which tend to be higher in protein and lower in fiber and poisons than mature leaves. Amongst humans, various food processing techniques are used worldwide to detoxify otherwise inedible foods and make them palatable.

Saltiness

Saltiness is a taste produced primarily by the

presence of sodium ions. Other ions of the alkali metals group also taste salty. However the further from sodium the less salty is the sensation. The size of lithium and potassium ions most closely resemble those of sodium and thus the saltiness is most similar. In contrast rubidium and cesium ions are far larger so their salty taste differs accordingly. The saltiness of substances is rated relative to sodium chloride (NaCl), which has an index of 1. Potassium, as potassium chloride - KCl, is the principal ingredient in salt substitutes, and has a saltiness index of 0.6.

Other monovalent cations, e.g. ammonium, NH_4+, and divalent cations of the alkali earth metal group of the periodic table, e.g. calcium, Ca_2+, ions generally elicit a bitter rather than a salty taste even though they too can pass directly through ion channels in the tongue, generating an action potential.

Sourness

Sourness is the taste that detects acidity. The sourness of substances is rated relative to dilute hydrochloric acid, which has a sourness index of 1. By comparison, tartaric acid has a sourness index of 0.7, citric acid an index of 0.46, and carbonic acid an index of 0.06. The mechanism for detecting sour taste is similar to that which detects salt taste. Hydrogen ion channels detect the concentration of hydronium ions (H_3O+ ions) that are formed from acids and water.

Hydrogen ions are capable of permeating the amiloride sensitive channels, but this is not the only mechanism involved in detecting the quality of sourness. Other channels have also been proposed in the literature. Hydrogen ions also inhibit the potassium channel, which normally functions to hyperpolarize the cell. By a combination of direct intake of hydrogen ions (which itself depolarizes the cell) and the inhibition of the hyperpolarizing channel, sourness causes the taste cell to fire in this specific manner. In addition, it has also been suggested that weak acids, such as CO2 which is converted into the bicarbonate ion HCO3− by the enzyme carbonic anhydrase, to mediate weak acid transport. The most common food group that contains naturally sour foods is the fruit, with examples such as the lemon, grape, orange, and sometimes the melon. Wine also usually has a sour tinge to its flavor. If not kept correctly, milk can spoil and contain a sour taste.

Sour candy is especially popular in North America including Cry babies, Warheads, lemon drops, and Shock Tarts.

Sweetness

Sweetness, usually regarded as a pleasurable sensation, is produced by the presence of sugars, some proteins and a few other substances. Sweetness is often connected to aldehydes and ketones, which contain a carbonyl group. Sweetness is detected by a variety of G protein coupled receptors coupled to the G protein gustducin found on the taste buds. At least two different variants of the "sweetness receptors" need to be activated for the brain to register sweetness. The compounds which the brain senses as sweet are thus compounds that can bind with varying bond strength to two different sweetness receptors. These receptors are T1R2+3 (heterodimer) and T1R3 (homodimer), which are shown to be accountable for all sweet sensing in humans and animals. Taste detection thresholds for sweet substances are rated relative to sucrose. The average human detection threshold for sucrose is 10 millimoles per litre. For lactose it is 30 millimoles per litre, with a sweetness index of 0.3[18], and 5-Nitro-2-propoxyaniline 0.002 millimoles per litre.

Umami

Umami is the name for the taste sensation produced by compounds such as glutamate, and are commonly found in fermented and aged foods. In English, it is also described as "meatiness", "relish", or "savoriness". The Japanese word comes from umai for delicious, keen, or nice. Umami is now the term commonly used by taste scientists. The same taste is referred to as xianwèi in Chinese cooking. Umami is considered a fundamental taste in Chinese and Japanese cooking, but is not discussed as much in Western cuisine.

Humans have taste receptors specifically for the detection of the amino acids, e.g., glutamic acid. Amino acids are the building blocks of proteins and are found in meats, cheese, fish, and other protein-heavy foods. Examples of food containing glutamate (and thus strong in umami) are beef, lamb, parmesan, and roquefort cheese as well as soy sauce and fish sauce. The glutamate taste sensation is most intense in combination with sodium ions, as found in table salt. Sauces with umami and salty tastes are very popular for cooking, such as worcestershire sauce for Western cuisines and soy sauce and fish sauce for Asian cuisines.

The additive monosodium glutamate (MSG), which was developed as a food additive in 1907 by Kikunae Ikeda, produces a strong umami. Umami is also provided by the nucleotides 5'-inosine monophosphate (IMP) and 5'-guanosine monophosphate (GMP). These are naturally present in many protein-rich foods. IMP is present in high concentrations in many foods, including dried skipjack tuna flakes used to make "dashi", a Japanese broth. GMP is present in high concentration in dried shiitake mushrooms, used in much of the cuisine of Asia. There is a synergistic effect between MSG, IMP, and GMP which together in certain ratios produce a strong umami.

Some umami taste buds respond specifically to glutamate in the same way that "sweet" ones respond to sugar. Glutamate binds to a variant of G protein coupled glutamate receptors.

OLFACTION

Olfaction (also known as olfactics or more commonly as smell) refers to the sense of smell. This sense is mediated by specialized sensory cells of the nasal cavity of vertebrates, and, by analogy, sensory cells of the antennae of invertebrates. For air-breathing animals, the olfactory system detects volatile or, in the case of the accessory olfactory system, fluid-phase chemicals. For water-dwelling organisms, e.g., fish or crustaceans, the chemicals are present in the surrounding aqueous medium. Olfaction, along with taste, is a form of chemoreception. The chemicals themselves which activate the olfactory system, generally at very low concentrations, are called odours.

OLFACTORY SYSTEM

Olfactory Epithelium

In vertebrates smells are sensed by olfactory sensory neurons in the olfactory epithelium. The proportion of olfactory epithelium compared to respiratory epithelium (not innervated) gives an indication of the animal's olfactory sensitivity. Humans have about 10 cm^2 of olfactory epithelium, whereas some dogs have 170 cm2. A dog's olfactory epithelium is also considerably more densely innervated, with a hundred times more receptors per square centimetre.

Molecules of odorants passing through the superior nasal concha of the nasal passages dissolve in the mucus lining the superior portion of the cavity and are detected

► Olfactory System

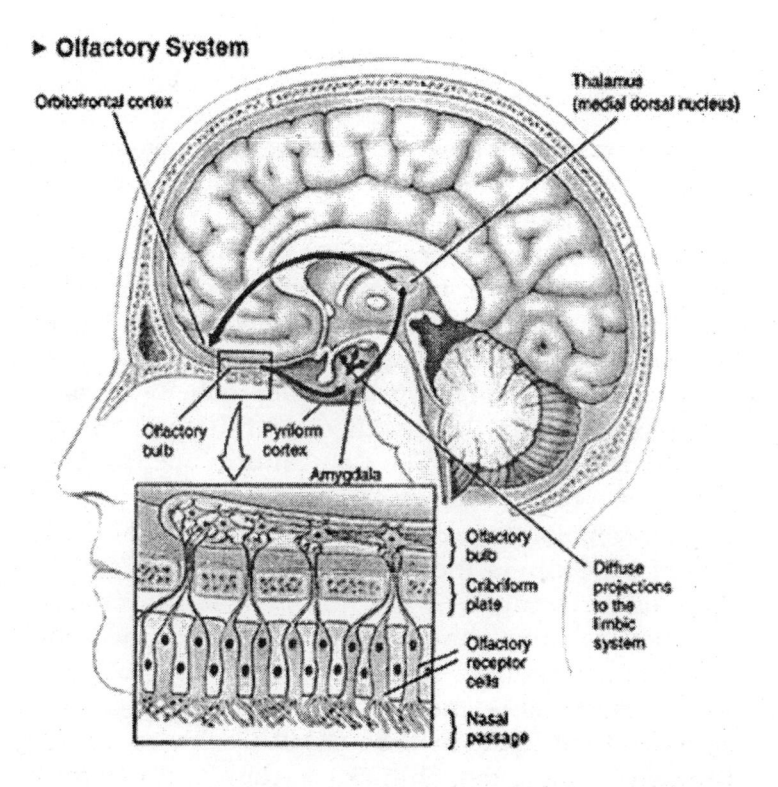

[Diagram of olfactory system showing: Orbitofrontal cortex, Thalamus (medial dorsal nucleus), Olfactory bulb, Pyriform cortex, Amygdala, Cribriform plate, Olfactory receptor cells, Nasal passage, Diffuse projections to the limbic system]

by olfactory receptors on the dendrites of the olfactory sensory neurons. This may occur by diffusion or by the binding of the odorant to odorant binding proteins. The mucus overlying the epithelium contains mucopolysaccharides, salts, enzymes, and antibodies (these are highly important, as the olfactory neurons provide a direct passage for infection to pass to the brain).

In insects smells are sensed by olfactory sensory neurons in the chemosensory sensilla, which are present in insect antenna, palps and tarsa, but also on other parts of the insect body. Odorants penetrate into the cuticle pores of chemosensory sensilla and get in contact with insect Odorant binding proteins (OBPs) or Chemosensory proteins (CSPs), before activating the sensory neurons.

Receptor Neuron

The process of how the binding of the ligand (odor molecule or odorant) to the receptor leads to an action potential in the receptor neuron is via a second messenger pathway depending on the organism. In mammals the odorants stimulate adenylate cyclase to synthesize cAMP via a G protein called Golf. cAMP, which is the second messenger here, opens a cyclic nucleotide-gated ion channel (CNG) producing an influx of cations (largely Ca^{2+} with some Na^+) into the cell, slightly depolarising it. The Ca^{2+} in turn opens a Ca^{2+}-activated chloride channel, leading to efflux of Cl^-, further depolarising the cell and triggering an action potential. Ca^{2+} is then extruded through a sodium-calcium exchanger. A calcium-calmodulin complex also acts to inhibit the binding of cAMP to the cAMP-dependent channel, thus contributing to olfactory adaptation. This mechanism of transduction is somewhat unique, in that cAMP works by directly binding to the ion channel rather than through activation of protein kinase A. It is similar to the transduction mechanism for photoreceptors, in which the second messenger cGMP works by directly binding to ion channels, suggesting that maybe one of these receptors was evolutionarily adapted into the other. There are also considerable similarities in the immediate processing of stimuli by lateral inhibition.

Averaged activity of the receptor neurons can be measured in several ways. In vertebrates responses to an odor can be measured by an electroolfactogram or through calcium imaging of receptor neuron terminals in the olfactory bulb. In insects, one can perform electroantenogram or also calcium imaging within the olfactory bulb.

The receptor neurons in the nose are particularly interesting because they are the only direct recipient of stimuli in all of the senses which are nerves. Senses like hearing, tasting, and, to some extent, touch use cilia or other indirect pressure to stimulate nerves, and sight uses the chemical Rhodopsin to stimulate the brain.

Olfactory Bulb Projections

Olfactory sensory neurons project axons to the brain within the olfactory nerve, (cranial nerve I). These axons pass to the olfactory bulb through the cribriform plate, which in turn projects olfactory information to the olfactory cortex and other areas. The axons from the olfactory receptors converge in the olfactory bulb within small (~50 micrometers in diameter) structures called glomeruli. Mitral cells in the olfactory bulb form synapses with the axons within glomeruli and send the information about the odor to multiple other parts of the olfactory system in the brain, where multiple signals may be processed to form a synthesized olfactory perception. There is a large degree of convergence here, with twenty-five thousand axons synapsing on one hundred or so mitral cells, and with each of these mitral cells projecting to multiple glomeruli. Mitral cells also project to periglomerular cells and granular cells that inhibit the mitral cells surrounding it (lateral inhibition). Granular cells also mediate inhibition and excitation of mitral cells through pathways from centrifugal fibres and the anterior olfactory nuclei.

The mitral cells leave the olfactory bulb in the lateral olfactory tract, which synapses on five major regions of the cerebrum: the anterior olfactory nucleus, the olfactory tubercle, the amygdala, the piriform cortex, and the entorhinal cortex. The anterior olfactory nucleus projects, via the anterior commissure, to the contralateral olfactory bulb, inhibiting it. The piriform cortex projects to the medial dorsal nucleus of the thalamus, which then projects to the orbitofrontal cortex. The orbitofrontal cortex mediates conscious perception of the odor. The 3-layered piriform cortex projects to a number of thalamic and hypothalamic nuclei, the hippocampus and amygdala and the orbitofrontal cortex but its function is largely unknown. The entorhinal cortex projects to the amygdala and is involved in emotional and autonomic responses to odor. It also projects to the hippocampus and is involved in motivation and memory. Odor information is easily stored in long-term memory and has strong connections to emotional memory. This is possibly due to the olfactory system's close anatomical ties to the limbic system and hippocampus, areas of the brain that have long been known to be involved in emotion and place memory, respectively.

Since any one receptor is responsive to various odorants, and there is a great deal of convergence at the level of the olfactory bulb, it seems strange that human beings are able to distinguish so many different odors. It seems that there must be a highly-complex form of processing occurring; however, as it can be shown that, while many neurons in the olfactory bulb (and even the pyriform cortex and amygdala) are responsive to many different odors, half the neurons in the orbitofrontal cortex are responsive only to one odor, and the rest to only a few. It has been shown through microelectrode studies that each individual odor gives a particular specific spatial map of excitation in the olfactory bulb. It is possible that, through spatial encoding, the brain is able to distinguish specific odors. However, temporal coding must be taken into account. Over time, the spatial maps change, even for one particular odour, and the brain must be able to process these details as well.

In insects smells are sensed by sensilla located on

the antenna and first processed by the antennal lobe (analogous to the olfactory bulb), and next by the mushroom bodies.

Pheromonal Olfaction

Many animals, including most mammals and reptiles, have two distinct and segregated olfactory systems: a main olfactory system, which detects volatile stimuli, and an accessory olfactory system, which detects fluid-phase stimuli. Behavioral evidence suggests that these fluid-phase stimuli often function as pheromones, although pheromones can also be detected by the main olfactory system. In the accessory olfactory system, stimuli are detected by the vomeronasal organ, located in the vomer, between the nose and the mouth. Snakes use it to smell prey, sticking their tongue out and touching it to the organ. Some mammals make a face called flehmen to direct air to this organ.

In women, the sense of olfaction is strongest around the time of ovulation, significantly stronger than during other phases of the menstrual cycle and also stronger than the sense in males.

The MHC genes (known as HLA in humans) are a group of genes present in many animals and important for the immune system; in general, offspring from parents with differing MHC genes have a stronger immune system. Fish, mice and female humans are able to smell some aspect of the MHC genes of potential sex partners and prefer partners with MHC genes different from their own.

Humans can detect individuals that are blood related kin (mothers and children but not husbands and wives) from olfaction. Mothers can identify by body odor their biological children but not their stepchildren. Preadolescent children can olfactory detect their full siblings but not half-siblings or step siblings and this might explain incest avoidance and the Westermarck effect. Functional imaging shows that this olfactory kinship detection process involves the frontal-temporal junction, the insula, and the dorsomedial prefrontal cortex but not the primary or secondary olfactory cortices, or the related piriform cortex or orbitofrontal cortex.

Olfaction and Taste

Olfaction, taste and trigeminal receptors together contribute to flavour. The human tongue can distinguish only among five distinct qualities of taste, while the nose can distinguish among hundreds of substances, even in minute quantities.

SOMATOSENSORY SYSTEM

The somatosensory system is a diverse sensory system comprising the receptors and processing centres to produce the sensory modalities such as touch, temperature, proprioception (body position), and nociception (pain). The sensory receptors cover the skin and epithelia, skeletal muscles, bones and joints, internal organs, and the cardiovascular system. While touch is considered one of the five traditional senses, the impression of touch is formed from several modalities; In medicine, the colloquial term touch is usually replaced with somatic senses to better reflect the variety of mechanisms involved.

The system reacts to diverse stimuli using different receptors: thermoreceptors, mechanoreceptors and chemoreceptors. Transmission of information from the receptors passes via sensory nerves through tracts in the spinal cord and into the brain. Processing primarily occurs in the primary somatosensory area in the parietal lobe of the cerebral cortex.

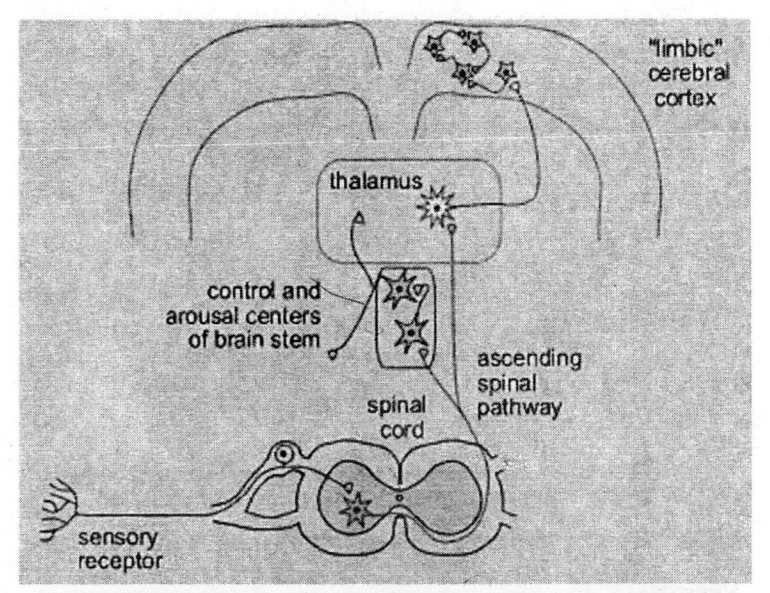

At its simplest, the system works when a sensory neuron is triggered by a specific stimulus such as heat; this neuron passes to an area in the brain uniquely attributed to that area on the body—this allows the processed stimulus to be felt at the correct location. The mapping of the body surfaces in the brain is called a homunculus and is essential in the creation of a body image.

Anatomy

The somatosensory system is spread through all major parts of a mammal's body (and other vertebrates). It consists both of sensory receptors and sensory (afferent) neurones in the periphery (skin, muscle and organs for example), to deeper neurones within the central nervous system.

General Somatosensory Pathway

A somatosensory pathway will typically has two long neurons: primary, secondary and tertiary (or first, second, and third).

The first neuron always has its cell body in the dorsal root ganglion of the spinal nerve (if sensation is in head or neck, it will be the trigeminal nerve ganglia or the ganglia of other sensory cranial nerves).

The second neuron has its cell body either in the spinal cord or in the brainstem. This neuron's ascending axons will cross (decussate) to the opposite side either in the spinal cord or in the brainstem. The axons of many of these neurones terminate in the thalamus (for example the ventral posterior nucleus, VPN), others terminate in the reticular system or the cerebellum.

In the case of touch and certain types of pain, the third neuron has its cell body in the VPN of the thalamus and ends in the postcentral gyrus of the parietal lobe.

Periphery

In the periphery, the somatosensory system detects various stimuli by sensory receptors, e.g. by mechanoreceptors for tactile sensation and nociceptors for pain sensation. The sensory information (touch, pain, temperature etc.,) is then conveyed to the central nervous system by afferent neurones. There are a number of different types of afferent neurones which vary in their size, structure and properties. Generally there is a correlation between the type of sensory modality detected and the type of afferent neurone involved. So for example slow, thin unmyelinated neurones conduct pain whereas faster, thicker, myelinated neurones conduct casual touch.

Spinal Cord

In the spinal cord, the somatosensory system includes ascending pathways from the body to the brain. One major target within the brain is the postcentral gyrus in the cerebral cortex. This is the target for neurones of the Dorsal Column Medial Lemniscal pathway and the Ventral Spinothalamic pathway. Note that many ascending somatosensory pathways include synapses in either the thalamus or the reticular formation before they reach the cortex. Other ascending pathways, particularly those involved with control of posture are projected to the cerebellum. These include the ventral and dorsal spinocerebellar tracts.

Brain

The primary somatosensory area in the human cortex is located in the postcentral gyrus of the parietal lobe. The postcentral gyrus is the location of the primary somatosensory area, the main sensory receptive area for the sense of touch. Like other sensory areas, there is a map of sensory space called a homunculus at this location. For the primary somatosensory cortex, this is called the sensory homunculus. Areas of this part of the human brain map to certain areas of the body, dependent on the amount or importance of somatosensory input from that area. For example, there is a large area of cortex devoted to sensation in the hands, while the back has a much smaller area. Interestingly, one study showed somatosensory cortex was found to be 21% thicker in 24 migraine sufferers, on average than in 12 controls[3], although we do not yet know what the significance of this is. Somatosensory information involved with proprioception and posture also targets an entirely different part of the brain, the cerebellum.

Touch Deprivation

Touch deprivation is when someone experiences an excessive lack in the sense of touch, often during the development in infancy, affecting the wellness of a person. Touch deprivation in infants leads to many different issues later in life. It affects the behavioral, health and physiological development of a human. With only minimal research in the field of touch deprivation, there is only a short history of the research and effects. Touch, before research conducted, was seen as only a minor impact of the development of a person. But according to an article by Robert Hatfield, Ph.D. from the University of Cincinnati, in 1945-1947, that view began to fall apart. Premature infants and sick toddlers were dying unexpectedly, so Dr. Rene Spitz, the caregiver, searched for explanation to the deaths. Not until 1958-1962, in Harry Harlow's research, was the mystery solved (Hatfield). The children were not being provided enough touch. Through Harlow's research with monkey infants he was able to discover the great importance of touch. Research following by John Bowlby and Mary Salter Ainsworth, confirmed the impact touch has on the attachment theory (Hatfield). Robert Hatfield discusses the results of these experiments and stated, "Affectionate touch vs. neglect or punishing touch is a central theme of Attachment Theory and much of this work may be viewed as the human research counterpart to the Harlow studies"

Physiology

Initiation of probably all "somatosensation" begins with activation of some sort of physical "receptor". These somatosensory receptors tend to lie in skin, organs or muscle. The structure of these receptors is broadly similar in all cases, consisting of either a "free nerve ending" or a nerve ending embedded in a specialised capsule. They can be activated by movement (mechanoreceptor), pressure (mechanoreceptor), chemical (chemoreceptor) and/or temperature. Another activation is by vibrations generated as a finger scans across a surface. This is the means by which we can sense fine textures in which the spatial scale is less than 200 μms. Such vibrations are around 250 Hz, which is the optimal frequency sensitivity of Pacinian corpuscles.

11

Reproductive System

The reproductive system is a system of organs within an organism which work together for the purpose of reproduction. Many non-living substances such as fluids, hormones, and pheromones are also important accessories to the reproductive system. Unlike most organ systems, the sexes of differentiated species often have significant differences. These differences allow for a combination of genetic material between two individuals, which allows for the possibility of greater genetic fitness of the offspring.

The major organs of the human reproductive system include the external genitalia (penis and vulva) as well as a number of internal organs including the gamete producing gonads (testicles and ovaries). Diseases of the human reproductive system are very common and widespread, particularly communicable sexually transmitted diseases.

Most other vertebrate animals have generally similar reproductive systems consisting of gonads, ducts, and openings. However, there is a great diversity of physical adaptations as well as reproductive strategies in every group of vertebrates.

MALE REPRODUCTIVE SYSTEM

The human male reproductive system is a series of organs located outside of the body and around the pelvic region of a male that contribute towards the reproductive process. The primary direct function of the male reproductive system is to provide the male gamete or spermatozoa for fertilization of the ovum.

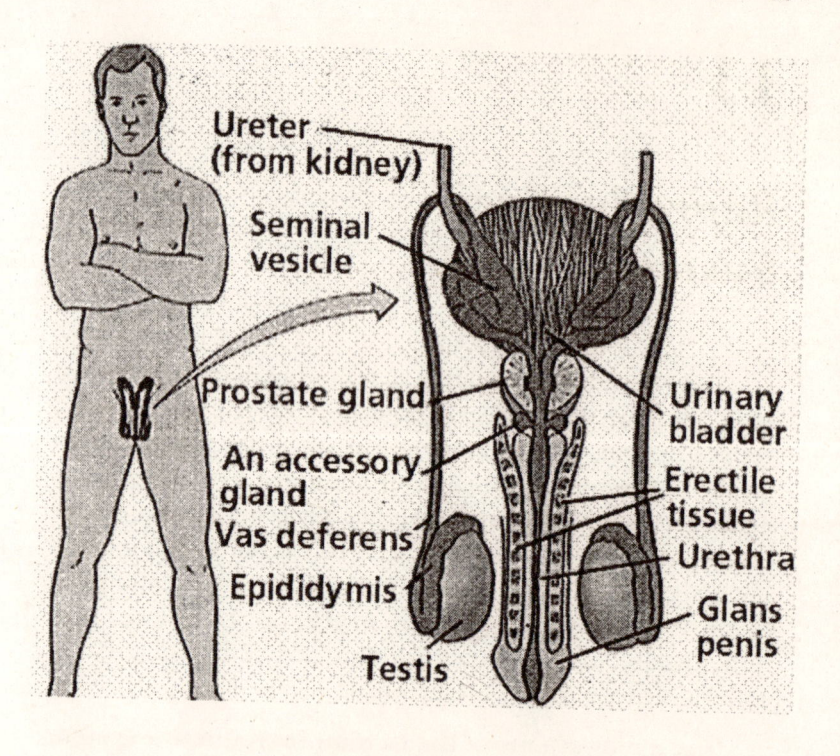

The major reproductive organs of the male can be grouped into three categories. The first category is sperm production and storage. Production takes place in the testes which are housed in the temperature regulating scrotum, immature sperm then travel to the epididymis for development and storage. The second category are the ejaculatory fluid producing glands which include the seminal vesicles, prostate, and the vas deferens. The final category are those used for copulation, and deposition of the spermatozoa (sperm) within the female, these include the penis, urethra, vas deferens, and Cowper's gland.

Reproductive System

Major secondary sexual characteristics include: larger, more muscular stature, deepened voice, facial and body hair, broad shoulders, and development of an adam's apple. An important sexual hormone of males is androgen, and particularly testosterone.

FEMALE REPRODUCTIVE SYSTEM

The human female reproductive system contains three main parts: the vagina, which acts as the receptacle for the male's sperm, the uterus, which holds the developing fetus, and the ovaries, which produce the female's ova. The breasts are also an important reproductive organ during the parenting stage of reproduction.

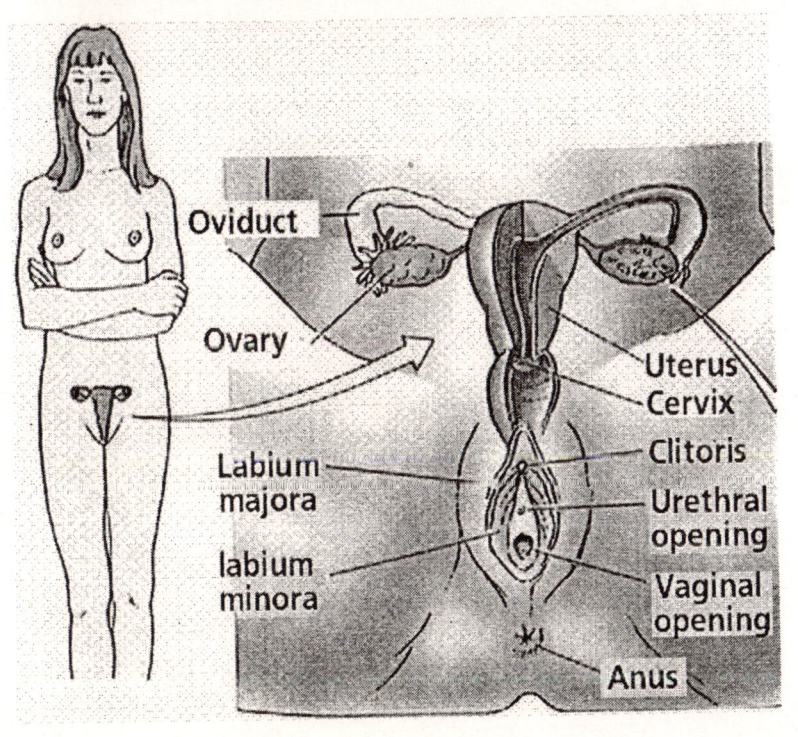

The vagina meets the outside at the vulva, which also includes the labia, clitoris and urethra; during intercourse this area is lubricated by mucus secreted by the Bartholin's glands. The vagina is attached to the uterus through the cervix, while the uterus is attached to the ovaries via the fallopian tubes. At certain intervals, typically approximately every 28 days, the ovaries release an ovum, which passes through the fallopian tube into the uterus. The lining of the uterus, called the endometrium, and unfertilized ova are shed each cycle through a process known as menstruation.

Major secondary sexual characteristics include: a smaller stature, a high percentage of body fat, wider hips, development of mammary glands, and enlargement of breasts. Important sexual hormones of females include estrogen and progesterone.

Production of Gametes

Main articles: Spermatogenesis and Oogenesis

The production of gametes takes place within the gonads through a process known as gametogenesis. Gametogenesis occurs when certain types of germ cells undergo meiosis to split the normal diploid number of chromosomes in humans (n=46) into haploids cells containing only 23 chromosomes.

In males this process is known as spermatogenesis and takes place only after puberty in the seminiferous tubules of the testes. The immature spermatozoon or sperm are then sent to the epididymis where they gain a tail and motility. Each of the original diploid germs cells or primary spermatocytes forms four functional gametes which is each capable of fertilization.

In females gametogenesis is known as oogenesis which occurs in the ovarian follicles of the ovaries. This process does not produce mature ovum until puberty. In contrast with males, each of the original diploid germ cells or primary oocytes will form only one mature ovum, and three polar bodies which are not capable of fertilization.

It has long been understood that in females, unlike males, all of the primary oocytes ever found in a female will be created prior to birth, and that the final stages of ova production will then not resume until puberty.[6] However, recent scientific data has challenged that hypothesis. This new data indicates that in at least some species of mammal oocytes continue to be replenished in females well after birth.

Development of the Reproductive System

The development of the reproductive system and urinary systems are closely tied in the development of the human fetus. Despite the differences between the adult male and female reproductive system, there are a number of homologous structures shared between them due to their common origins within the fetus. Both organ systems are derived from the intermediate mesoderm. The three main fetal precursors of the reproductive organs are the Wolffian duct, Müllerian ducts, and the gonad. Endocrine hormones are a well known and critical controlling factor in the normal differentiation of the reproductive system.

The Wolffian duct forms the epididymis, vas deferns, ductus deferens, ejaculatory duct, and seminal vesicle in the male reproductive system and essentially disappears in the female reproductive system. For the Müllerian Duct this process is reversed as it essentially disappears in the male reproductive system and forms the fallopian tubes uterus, and vagina in the female system. In both sexes the gonad goes on to form the testes and ovaries, because they are derived from the same undeveloped structure they are considered homologous organs. There are a number of other homologous structures shared between male and female reproductive systems. However, despite the similarity in function of the female fallopian tubes and the male epididymis and vas deferens, they are not homologous but rather analogous structures as they arise from different fetal structures.

12

Physiology of Exercise

Exercise physiology is the study of the function of the human body during various acute and chronic exercise conditions. These effects are significant during both short, high intensity exercise as well as with prolonged strenuous exercise such as done in endurance sports like marathons, ultramarathons, and road bicycle racing.

In exercise, the liver generates extra glucose, while increased cardiovascular activity by the heart, and respiration by the lungs, provides an increased supply of oxygen. When exercise is very prolonged and strenuous, a decline, however, can occur in blood levels of glucose. In some individuals, this might even cause hypoglycemia and hypoxemia. There can also be cognitive and physical impairments due to dehydration. Another risk is low plasma sodium blood levels.

Prolonged exercise is made possible by the human thermoregulation capacity to remove exercise waste heat by sweat evaporation. This capacity evolved to enable early humans after many hours of persistence hunting to exhaust game animals that cannot remove so effectively exercise heat from their body.

EFFECT OF EXERCISE ON CIRCULATORY SYSTEM

Exercise produces a beneficial "training effect" on the entire cardiovascular system. The heart's pumping muscle, the skeletal muscles (movement muscles), the blood vessels and the red blood cells all grow in size or number with exercise. These gradual changes are all geared towards transporting more blood (oxygen and nutrients) to the body and then efficiently removing waste (carbon dioxide and, importantly, heat) away from the body. There are two major categories of exercise, and each creates a slightly different training effect. Resistance exercise (lifting weights for example) tends to make the heart muscle (left ventricular pumping chamber) somewhat thicker without changing the volume of blood contained in the heart so much. Endurance or "aerobic" type exercises (running and swimming for example) increase muscle strength and stamina but the muscles do not enlarge as much as they would with resistance exercise. Endurance exercises cause the heart's left ventricle pumping chamber size to gradually increase in volume over time. This training effect allows that heart muscle to pump more blood to the body with each beat and with less effort. Exercise also causes a growth in the number of small blood vessels (arterioles and capillaries) that supply the skeletal muscles. Regular vigorous exercise causes the body to produce more oxygen-containing red blood cells as well. This explains why regular "aerobic" endurance training greatly improves the "huffing and puffing" that can come from normal activities such as climbing stairs. With each breath, there are more blood vessels that are filled with more red blood cells pumped by a larger heart so that oxygen taken in with each breath is more quickly and efficiently delivered where it is needed.

In summary, regular vigorous exercise produces a training effect by "remodeling" the body's entire cardiovascular system over time. This explains why physical fitness training is a gradual process that requires patience. Ultimately the benefits of regular exercise are enormous. A person who exercises vigorously and regularly has lower levels of circulating stress-related hormones and this improves the health of the blood vessel lining. This reduces the chance of plaque build up which can cause heart attack or stroke. Not being "stressed out" by everyday activities also creates an improved sense of well being and the ability to more quickly bounce back from injuries or surgical procedures. Unfortunately, "detraining" happens more quickly than the training process. Exercise must be continued daily or at least on alternate days to maintain a level of fitness. Most athletes know all too well how much ground can be lost after even 2 or 3 weeks off of training and the heart's size can be shown to shrink back to baseline in this short of a period of time. It is a good idea to combine both endurance and resistance exercises and many sports are, in fact, a combination of these. The most important thing is to find a way to have fun during exercise so that it can be looked forward to as part of a normal "lifestyle." This will lead to the best long-term cardiovascular health.

EFFECT OF EXERCISE ON RESPIRATORY SYSTEM

Training effect is the elevation of metabolism through physical exercise. This effect was discovered by Dr. Kenneth H. Cooper for the United States Air Force in the late 1960s. Dr. Cooper coined the term "Training Effect" for this.

The measured effects were that muscles of respiration were strengthened, the heart was strengthened, blood pressure was sometimes lowered and the total amount of blood and number of red blood cells increased, making the blood a more efficient carrier of oxygen. VO_2 Max was increased.

The exercise necessary can be accomplished by any aerobic exercise in a wide variety of schedules - Dr. Cooper found it best to award "points" for each amount of exercise (as laid out in the detailed tables in his classic 1968 book "Aerobics", reprinted and expanded several times) and require 30 points a week to maintain the Training Effect.

Dr. Cooper instead recommended a "12-minute test" (the Cooper test) followed by adherence to the appropriate starting-up schedule in his book. As always, he recommends that a physical exam should precede any exercise program. (A newly-recognized effect is that of Exercise hypertension, for which there is a medical test.)

The physiological effects of training have received much further study since Dr. Cooper's original work. It is now generally considered that effects of exercise on general metabolic rate (post-exercise) are comparatively small and the greatest effect occurs for only a few hours. However, all exercise components (summarised perhaps as general endurance - as reflected to a degree by VO_2 max, strength, local muscular endurance, and flexibility) are significantly trainable at all ages in many people, and the Cooper Points System still gives overall guidance on this.

The effects of exercise on the respiratory system

Short Term Effects

During exercise, the body needs a supply of oxygen to release energy in the muscles.

Respiration increases to provide that oxygen and remove carbon dioxide.

This is done by:

• increasing breathing rate by about three times the normal rate.

• increasing tidal volume by five times the normal

rate.
- increasing blood supply to and through the lungs.
- increasing oxygen up take.

Note: Tidal Volume is the amount of air taken in or out with each breathe.

Long Term Effects

The body becomes more efficient at using oxygen.

This is known as VO_2 max and is a significant indicator of an athlete's physical fitness.

VO_2 max can be accurately tested.

EFFECT OF EXERCISE ON DIGESTIVE SYSTEM

Short Term Effects

- Blood is diverted to the heart, lungs and working muscles, away from parts of the digestive system.
- It is best to rest for up to two hours after a meal before exercising.

THE EFFECTS OF EXERCISE ON THE BODY

Short Term Effects

- During intense exercise the body's temperature rises.
- Messages are sent from the brain to the skin to make it sweat. Sweat is formed by sweat glands under the skin.
- Losing heat through sweating is caused by the evaporation of sweat from the skins surface.
- Blood is diverted to the capillaries just below the skin. This causes the skin to redden.

Long Term Effects

• Exercise improves the general health and well being of the body.

• It is kept toned and helps to prevent heart disease in later life.

• It provides positive mental and social contributions to a persons life as well as positive physical contributions.

EFFECT OF EXERCISE ON SKELETAL SYSTEM

Exercising tires the skeletal muscles. To make your skeletal muscles stronger and to make them tire less quickly, you can practice using those muscles daily to build up strength.

Skeletal muscle is a complex organ composed of particular cells, multinucleate syncytia gathered in a connective network that peripherally continues with the tendinous structures necessary to transmit contractile force of muscle fibers on bone. Skeletal muscle is composed of heterogeneous fiber types that vary in contraction velocity, endurance capability and metabolic enzyme profile. Both vascular and nervous factors are particularly important for motor performance.

The management of the contractile machinery gathered inside myofibers is strictly linked to the activity of the myonuclei, mitochondria, and the system of T tubules and sarcoplasmic reticulum (SR). The way structural elements of myofibers are gathered strictly depends on the cytoskeletic system peripherally associated with the sarcolemma because of specific membrane proteins whose physiological role is to provide mechanical stability to the surface membrane during normal contraction as well as to carry out important receptor functions.

Skeletal muscle is a highly plastic tissue that adapts to changing functional demands by altering its constituent proteins. It is well established that strength training increases muscle strength and this increase is due to both neural and muscular factors. Chronic contractile activity in muscle, not otherwise subjected to such a stimulus, promotes changes in the complement of contractile and metabolic proteins that optimize muscle function for this new type of activity. Such remodelling involves altered patterns of both protein synthesis and protein degradation, thus making muscle tissue capable of enduring subsequent periods of exercise. Therefore, correct physical exercise involves several adaptations improving structural organization of both muscle and contractile performance. It is also true that strenuous exercise and particularly eccentric contraction (EC) determines the muscle damage reported in literature.

Effects of Exercise on Skeletal Muscle

Previously reported postexercise degenerative response includes an increase in fibrous connective tissue fiber necrosis, damage of contractile components, and disruption of membranous components, such as mitochondria. After exercise, the cytoskeletal network is damaged as a result of sarcolemmal disruption, occuring even before the alteration of the contractile components, thus representing one of the first targets hit by overload or total load absence. Such damage can be explained through alteration of the cytoskeletal anchoring system to the sarcolemma. This system involves different proteic complexes and particularly, the integrin and dystrophin-glycoprotein complexes

(DGC) that, as mentioned above, – mechanically match extra- and intracellular areas and work as membrane receptors activating a number of signalling systems towards the nuclei. Such systems are important because their absence or hypoexpression brings about serious muscular pathologies known as dystrophies. Immediately after exercise, some of the proteins belonging to these complexes decrease both quantitatively and qualitatively. This decrease is followed by a subsequent return to normal values after a few weeks and may provide a structural explanation for the protective effects towards a further series of exercises. It has been hypothesized that a repetition of eccentric exercise makes the extracellular matrix, myofibrils, cytoskeleton, and cell membranes more resistant, providing a morphological mechanism for rapid adaptation.

Statistical analyses of gene-exercise interactions and laboratory studies of cellular function have also revealed genes that are directly altered by exercise. Nevertheless, the mechanisms by which these alterations in gene expression subsequent to exercise occur have not been well studied.

Ultrastructural Changes

Acute and chronic exercise is associated with ultrastructural muscle damage that is mainly centered on the Z disk that anchors thin filaments and several intermediate filaments within the sarcomere. Most of the evidence pointing to Z-disk involvement comes from electron microscopic studies that show eccentric damaged sarcomeres, particularly sarcomeres out of register with one another, these disorganized sarcomeres coexisting with normal sarcomeres. Z disks appear to widen or disintegrate, and it is also possible to see regional disorganization of the myofilament and ttubule damage. Disturbances of the mitochondria, sarcoplasmic reticulum, A band, and extracellular matrix have also been reported. A common feature of after-training muscle fibers is the separation of myofibrils. It has been postulated that this separation may be indicative of damage to intermediate filament proteins such as desmin.

The ultrastructural disruptions of muscle fibers, such as the breakage of exosarcomeric cytoskeleton proteins or the distortion of the alignment of the A and I band in the absence of fibre degeneration, may affect the relationship between the basal lamina and satellite cells and induce the release of some growth factors known to affect satellite cell activation and proliferation, such as fibroblast growth factor or insulin growth factor. These cells, first identified by Mauro, are uniformly distributed throughout the length of the muscle and located between the basal lamina and sarcolemma. It has been demonstrated that short or long-term strength training can induce their activation.

A few weeks after EC, examination of muscle samples shows a normal ultrastructural myofibrillar profile, indicating the existence of a remodelling response after exercise-induced damage. This observation shows that the contractile machinery first damaged by exercise can recover and adapt to further overload.

Cytoskeletal Proteins

In addition to contractile proteins, muscle contains cytoskeletal proteins that stabilize the contractile proteins and allow for transmission of tension both longitudinally and laterally. These cytoskeleton proteins may have a role in the prevention or development of eccentric damage. Besides these, desmin, a protein of cell-matrix connection system, could be involved in the sarcomere disruption following eccentric exercise. Desmin is a structural protein located in the Z disks, connecting adjacent Z disks and Z disks at the edge of the fiber to the costamere in the surface membrane.

Thus it contributes to the alignment of Z disks across the fibers and also transmits lateral tension. Previous studies showed a loss of desmin immediately after EC. Such loss resulted from raised resting [Ca^{2+}]i but preceded damage to contractile proteins. Many desmin negative fibers showed normal contractile filaments so this may reflect different speeds of propagation of desmin loss and contractile filament disruption along the fibers. The mechanism by which loss of desmin staining occurs is not known; however, modifications in this staining could not be mediated by mechanisms that rely on gene regulation, but instead by mechanisms involving muscle fiber membrane disruption and subsequent proteolysis or conformational change of the cytoskeletal network. Finally, after the intermediate filaments are disrupted by an increase in [Ca^{2+}]i, that in turn activates proteasis [Ca^{2+}]i dependent such as calpain, the myofibrillar apparatus is disrupted and is unable to develop normal tension. The rapid loss of desmin, immediately after a single bout of eccentric contraction, recovers after 3-4 days, and such increase represents a remodelling of the intermediate filament system. Newly synthesized desmin could serve to reinforce existing sarcomeres or be added to newly synthesized sarcomeres. There is evidence suggesting the involvement of the small heat shock proteins (Hsp) in the process of remodelling, particularly in the assembly and maintenance of the intermediate filament network.

Hsp are important components of the cellular protective response against reactive oxygen species (ROS) and recent data indicate an increase in the expression of numerous Hsps in response to exercise and endurance training.

Previous studies report that cytoskeleton disruption occurred as fast as 5 min. after initiation of EC; such results suggest that direct mechanical or biochemical events are responsible for this disruption, rather than events that require gene regulation.

The main system of the cellular-matrix interaction systems is represented by two receptor complexes: dystrophin associated glycoproteins and integrins associated to talin and vinculin. Recently, a study carried out on human skeletal muscle undergoing EC showed changes in the dystrophin-glycoprotein complex, in particular discontinuous staining for dystrophin and reduced expression of á-sarcoglycan immediately after EC. Thus, this loss may destabilize the sarcolemma leading to modifications of membrane permeability. The decrease in the level of a-sarcoglycan may also regulate the intracellular calcium concentration and therefore, lead to the persistent activation of P2X receptors, resulting in intracellular [Ca2+]i overloaded in muscle fibres that in turn may activate [Ca2+]i -dependent proteolitic pathways. This loss occurs before the loss of staining of the cytoskeletal protein desmin or before the staining of disorganized actin and may have an origin in the disruption of the plasma membrane. The subsequent recovery of these proteic complexes after a few weeks may be involved in the subsequent remodelling of myofibrillar structure and this response may limit the extent of muscle damage upon a subsequent mechanical stress.

A single bout of moderate eccentric exercise leads to profound adaptations in human skeletal muscle; the specific mechanisms involved in this response have yet to be determined. However, from proteolytic response data, the differential expression of structural proteins and the induction of molecular chaperons appear to be involved in the damage-repair process.

Excitation-Contraction Coupling

Eccentric exercise may have effects on excitationcontraction coupling, possibly affecting both the release and uptake of [Ca2+]i by the sarcoplasmic reticulum. It has been shown that downhill running exercise results in changes in the organization of the membrane system involved in E-C coupling in skeletal muscle fibers. The arrangement of the t-tubule network and the disposition of the triads changed following downhill running exercise. Several authors have shown that intracellular [Ca2+]i accumulation causes muscle damage and since membrane depolarization is associated with [Ca2+]i release from the SR, it is possible that repeated muscle contractions combined with impaired [Ca2+]i uptake by the SR lead to muscle degeneration.

Conclusions

It is clear that eccentric exercise causes a number of ultrastructural, biochemical and metabolic alterations that at first glance appear to be devastating to the integrity of the muscle. Indeed, when physical exercise is occasional and intense, especially in sedentary and elderly subjects, muscle integrity is compromised. The mechanical damage induced by moderate and continuous exercise – specific to regular training – turns out to be a positive condition in that it can bring about structural and metabolic remodelling capable of increasing endurance towards subsequent mechanical stress. This capacity of adaptation is also associated with numerous changes in gene expression, upregulation of cellular protective mechanisms, and remodelling of muscle structure. Several factors can determine modifications of the gene expression and many of the signalling systems that can induce such changes are well known (autocrine, paracrine, hormonal, neural, growth factors, intermediate metabolite flows, etc.). Most of these signalling systems have myonuclei as targets because they can modify their processes of translation and transcription of mRNA. It has been recently suggested that the mechanical forces which develop during training can also directly influence the function of myonuclei through the stimulation of the membrane proteins associated with the cytoskeleton.

Depending on the intensity and amount of the applied stimulus, striated muscle can undergo 1) remodelling of its contractile machinery, 2) changes of neuromuscular junction, 3) changes of [Ca2+]i release and in the [Ca2+]i sensitivity of the contractile machinery; 4) upregulation of the mitochondrial system, 5) possible myonuclei increase through activation of satellite cells, 6) increases in its capillarity and blood flow/oxygen utilization capacity.

Many of these changes can be ascribed to the release of important regulation factors among which nitric oxide (NO) plays a key role. Its production in muscle is increased by exercise as a result of the chronic inflammation caused by training.